CARDIOLOGY RESEARCH AND CLINICAL DEVELOPMENTS

CARDIOMETABOLIC DISEASES AND RISK FACTORS

CARDIOLOGY RESEARCH AND CLINICAL DEVELOPMENTS

Additional books and e-books in this series can be found on Nova's website under the Series tab.

CARDIOLOGY RESEARCH AND CLINICAL DEVELOPMENTS

CARDIOMETABOLIC DISEASES AND RISK FACTORS

PATRICK RALSTON
EDITOR

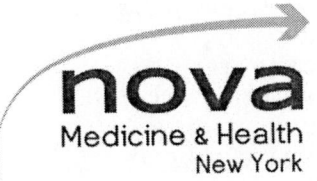

Copyright © 2020 by Nova Science Publishers, Inc.

All rights reserved. No part of this book may be reproduced, stored in a retrieval system or transmitted in any form or by any means: electronic, electrostatic, magnetic, tape, mechanical photocopying, recording or otherwise without the written permission of the Publisher.

We have partnered with Copyright Clearance Center to make it easy for you to obtain permissions to reuse content from this publication. Simply navigate to this publication's page on Nova's website and locate the "Get Permission" button below the title description. This button is linked directly to the title's permission page on copyright.com. Alternatively, you can visit copyright.com and search by title, ISBN, or ISSN.

For further questions about using the service on copyright.com, please contact:
Copyright Clearance Center
Phone: +1-(978) 750-8400   Fax: +1-(978) 750-4470   E-mail: info@copyright.com.

NOTICE TO THE READER

The Publisher has taken reasonable care in the preparation of this book, but makes no expressed or implied warranty of any kind and assumes no responsibility for any errors or omissions. No liability is assumed for incidental or consequential damages in connection with or arising out of information contained in this book. The Publisher shall not be liable for any special, consequential, or exemplary damages resulting, in whole or in part, from the readers' use of, or reliance upon, this material. Any parts of this book based on government reports are so indicated and copyright is claimed for those parts to the extent applicable to compilations of such works.

Independent verification should be sought for any data, advice or recommendations contained in this book. In addition, no responsibility is assumed by the Publisher for any injury and/or damage to persons or property arising from any methods, products, instructions, ideas or otherwise contained in this publication.

This publication is designed to provide accurate and authoritative information with regard to the subject matter covered herein. It is sold with the clear understanding that the Publisher is not engaged in rendering legal or any other professional services. If legal or any other expert assistance is required, the services of a competent person should be sought. FROM A DECLARATION OF PARTICIPANTS JOINTLY ADOPTED BY A COMMITTEE OF THE AMERICAN BAR ASSOCIATION AND A COMMITTEE OF PUBLISHERS.

Additional color graphics may be available in the e-book version of this book.

Library of Congress Cataloging-in-Publication Data

ISBN: 978-1-53618-111-1
Identifiers: LCCN 2020025128 (print) | LCCN 2020025129 (ebook) | ISBN
  9781536181111 (paperback) | ISBN 9781536181128 (adobe pdf)
Subjects: LCSH: Cardiovascular system--Diseases--Risk factors. |
  Metabolism--Disorders--Risk factors.
Classification: LCC RC669 .C2746 2020 (print) | LCC RC669 (ebook) | DDC
  616.1/071--dc23
LC record available at https://lccn.loc.gov/2020025128
LC ebook record available at https://lccn.loc.gov/2020025129

Published by Nova Science Publishers, Inc. † New York

CONTENTS

Preface		vii
Chapter 1	Cardiometabolic Diseases and Risk Factors *Fava Marie Claire, Agius Rachel and Fava Stephen*	1
Chapter 2	Cardio-Metabolic Risk Factors in Polycystic Ovary Syndrome *Fahimeh Ramezani Tehrani and Samira Behboudi-Gandevani*	43
Chapter 3	Cardiometabolic Risks Related to Obesity: Potential Effects of Nutritional Habits *Danielle Cristina Seiva, Yasmin Alaby Martins Ferreira, Marcos Mônico-Neto, Hanna Karen Moreira Antunes and Raquel Munhoz da Silveira Campos*	87
Index		117

PREFACE

In this compilation, the pathogenesis and interrelationships of metabolic abnormalities are discussed, particularly their impact on cardiovascular disease, as well as the role of excess adiposity in metabolic derange.

The authors discuss the literature on polycystic ovary syndrome and cardio-metabolic risk factors, providing recommendations that would be helpful for healthcare providers and policy makers.

Additionally, the aspects of nutritional habits associated to an increase in cardiovascular risk factors in the obese population are addressed. (Imprint: Nova Medicine and Health)

Chapter 1 - Metabolic derangements are a major driver of cardiovascular disease, which is in turn a major cause of mortality and morbidity. Important metabolic abnormalities include hyperinsulinaemia/insulin resistance, hypertriglyceridaemia, high circulating free fatty acids, low and dysfunctional high-density lipoprotein, production of small, dense low-density lipoprotein and of oxidised low-density lipoprotein, and dysglycaemia. Excess adiposity is one of the major drivers for metabolic unhealthliness which is growing global public health problem paralleling the pandemic of excessive adiposity.

In this review, the authors discuss the pathogenesis and inter-relationships of these metabolic abnormalities, their impact on cardiovascular disease as well as the role of excess adiposity in metabolic derangements. The authors also discuss the concept of metabolic health. The association of metabolic abnormalities with carcinogenesis is beyond the scope of this review.

Chapter 2 - Polycystic ovary syndrome (PCOS) is one of the most common endocrine disorders with an estimated prevalence of 7% to14% among reproductive-aged women. Although the exact underlying etiology of PCOS is not entirely clear, however, evidence has shown that insulin resistance, hyperandrogenemia and adipose tissue dysregulation play key roles on its pathogenesis. The syndrome is recognized as a cardio-metabolic disorder. Data have shown that traditional cardiovascular and metabolic risk factors including hypertension, dyslipidemia, metabolic syndrome, obesity and central obesity, glucose intolerance and diabetes are more prevalent among PCOS patients. In addition, subclinical cardiovascular markers such as coronary artery calcium scores, C-reactive protein, carotid intima-media thickness and endothelial dysfunction are more likely to be increased in women with PCOS. Nevertheless, there is much more controversy regarding whether cardio-metabolic events are increased in PCOS in later life, leaving many issues regarding cardiovascular and metabolic events unresolved. This chapter will discuss the literature on PCOS and cardio-metabolic risk factors and provides recommendations that would be helpful for healthcare provider and policy makers in the monitoring and management of these risk factors in PCOS population. Treatment options are beyond the scope of this chapter.

Chapter 3 - Obesity is considerate a global epidemic with alarming consequences. Epidemiology data indicate that approximately 2.1 billion of adult population has obesity diagnosis. Data from World Health Organization demonstrated that 36.20% in the United States, 27.80% in the United Kingdom and 22.10% in Brazil adult population were obese. Obesity is a multifactorial disease related to increase of body fat mass, metabolic disorders and a pro-inflammatory state. This framework induces to development of many comorbidities, including dyslipidemia, metabolic syndrome, non-alcoholic fatty liver disease and increase the cardiovascular risk factors. Considering the cardiovascular diseases (CDVs), it represents the number 1 cause of death in the world. Mostly of the CVDs can be prevented by lifestyle changes, for example, increase the physical activity and improve the nutritional habits. Specially for diet habits, this is an area who has aroused a relevant interesting, since nutritional behavior is an important strategy to prevent and treat several diseases. In fact, the impact of nutrition habits in obesity and CVDs was expensively studied. Although, recently the pro/anti-inflammatory effects of diet aroused interest from the scientific community, suggesting that foods can exert influence in metabolism pathway and be able to contribute or prevent the disease development, as obesity and cardiovascular diseases. In this way, the dietary inflammatory score was development to characterize the pro/anti-inflammatory effects of individuals diet and permitted to explore the possible associations with metabolic alterations related to several disease. In this sense, the present chapter will be exploring the aspects of nutritional habits and diet quality in the mechanism associated to increase on cardiovascular risk factors in obese population.

In: Cardiometabolic Diseases and Risk Factors ISBN: 978-1-53618-111-1
Editor: Patrick Ralston © 2020 Nova Science Publishers, Inc.

Chapter 1

CARDIOMETABOLIC DISEASES AND RISK FACTORS

Fava Marie Claire[1], *Agius Rachel*[1,2] *and Fava Stephen*[1,2,*]

[1]University of Malta, Msida, Malta
[2]Mater Dei Hospital, Msida, Malta

ABSTRACT

Metabolic derangements are a major driver of cardiovascular disease, which is in turn a major cause of mortality and morbidity. Important metabolic abnormalities include hyperinsulinaemia/insulin resistance, hypertriglyceridaemia, high circulating free fatty acids, low and dysfunctional high-density lipoprotein, production of small, dense low-density lipoprotein and of oxidised low-density lipoprotein, and dysglycaemia. Excess adiposity is one of the major drivers for metabolic unhealthliness which is growing global public health problem paralleling the pandemic of excessive adiposity.

In this review, we discuss the pathogenesis and inter-relationships of these metabolic abnormalities, their impact on cardiovascular disease as

---

[*] Corresponding Author's Email: stephen.fava@um.edu.mt.

well as the role of excess adiposity in metabolic derangements. We also discuss the concept of metabolic health. The association of metabolic abnormalities with carcinogenesis is beyond the scope of this review.

IMPORTANCE OF CARDIOVASCULAR DISEASE

Although there has been a decline in mortality from cardiovascular disease (CVD), it still remains a major public health problem (Rawshani A et al., 2017). One study has shown that CVD accounted for approximately 7.4 million deaths worldwide in 2012 which translates to 13.2% of total global deaths (McAloon CJ et al., 2016). It has also been shown that patients over 50 years of age with CVD live on average 7.8 years less than the general population (van Kruijsdijk RC et al., 2016). Mortality from cardiovascular disease is equivalent to the combined number of deaths due to nutritional deficiencies, infectious diseases, and maternal and perinatal conditions (Organization WH and UNAIDS).

CVD also puts a significant financial burden on health care systems and has significant societal costs. This is attributed to drug treatment, use of devices, health care consultations and loss of productivity particularly in people of working age (Balbay Y et al., 2018; Lakić D et al., 2014; National Center for Cardiovascular Diseases of China, 2017). This higherin those suffering from diabetes (Mehta S et al., 2018). Costs vary from country to country, but it has been estimated that the average cost is 6,466 US$ for unstable angina, 11,664 US$ for acute myocardial infarction, 11,686 US$ for acute heart failure, 13,501 US$ for percutaneous coronary intervention and 37,611 US$ for coronary artery bypass graft and (Nicholson G et al., 2016).

INSULIN RESISTANCE/HYPERINSULINAEMIA

Hyperinsulinaemia has been shown to predict cardiovascular disease. In the landmark Helsinki Policemen study (Pyorala M et al., 1998), an oral glucose tolerance test was performed on a cohort of 970 men who were free of CVD and diabetes at baseline, with blood glucose and plasma insulin measurements at 0, 1, and 2 hours. The study found that the area under the insulin curve during the oral glucose tolerance test was predictive of 22-year coronary heart disease events. Similarly fasting and 2-hour post-load plasma insulin levels were found to be independent predictors of coronary heart disease deaths after 11 years of follow-up in the Paris Prospective Study (Fontbonne AM et al., 1991). A meta-analysis by Hu G et al. (2004) found that fasting insulin levels are independently associated with CVD mortality in both men and women. C-peptide, which is co-secreted with insulin and serves as a marker of hyperinsulinaemia, has likewise been associated with increased CVD mortality (Marx N et al., 2013; Min JY et al., 2013). The fact that increased cardiovascular risk predates the onset of diabetes (Hu FB et al., 2002) makes likely that the increased risk associated with diabetes is at least partly attributable to preceding insulin resistance/hyperinsulinaemia.

At a cellular level, insulin exerts its effects through two distinct pathways. The metabolic and vasodilatory effects of insulin are mediated by the insulin receptor substrate-1/protein kinase B (IRS-1/AKT) pathway (Montagnani M et al., 2002). On the other hand, the mitogen-activated protein kinase (MAPK) pathway mediates the release of endothelin-1 and plasminogen activator inhibitor-1 (PAI-1) as well as the mitogenic properties of insulin (King GL et al., 2016). Insulin resistance is usually restricted to the IRS-1/AKT pathway. In insulin resistant states there is compensatory hyperinsulinaemia in an attempt to maintain euglycaemia. However, the hyperinsulinaemia drives overactivity of the MAPK pathway since this pathway is not resistant to the effects of insulin (King GL et al., 2016; Muniyappa R et al., 2013). The resultant imbalance between the two pathways leads to endothelial dysfunction, myocardial hypertrophy, cardiac fibrosis, and death of myocardial and endothelial cells. These changes predispose to both atherosclerosis and non-coronary artery disease mediated cardiac dysfunction (often referred to as 'diabetic cardiomyopathy') (Witteles RM et al., 2008; Falcao-Pires I et al., 2012; Mandavia CH et al., 2013). The increased mitogenicity associated with increased activity of the MAPK pathway probably also contributes to increased risk of malignancy associated with insulin resistant states, but this is beyond the scope of this review and is discussed elsewhere.

DYSGLYCAEMIA

Diabetes mellitus is a well-recognised risk factor for cardiovascular disease. In the Framingham study, diabetes emerged as an important risk factor even after adjusting for other traditional risk factors (Garcia MJ et al., 1974). In a meta-analysis of 37 prospective cohort studies with a total of 447,064 patients, Huxley R et al., (2006) reported that diabetes conferred an age-adjusted relative risk of coronary artery disease (CAD) mortality of 2.16 in men and of 3.69 in women. Peters SAE et al. (2014) have likewise confirmed that the relative risk associated with diabetes is greater in females than in males; women with diabetes are therefore said to lose their 'female advantage' with regard to CAD. The Emerging Risk Factors Collaboration (2010) reported an even larger meta-analysis than the one by Huxley at al. It included 102 prospective studies, 698,782 subjects and 8.49 million person-years at risk. It found that diabetes conferred doubling of CAD risk (an adjusted hazard ratio of 2.0). Finally, in the Multiple Risk Factor Intervention Trial [MRFIT] (Stamler J et al., 1993) diabetes was found to be associated the same risk as the combination of any other two risk factors. It is important to note that the risk is increased similarly in both type 1 and type 2 diabetes (Juutilainen et al. 2008). There is also a higher short-term (Fava S et al., 1993) and- long-term (up to 16 years) (Gruppetta M et al., 2010) mortality after myocardial infarction (MI) in subjects with type 2 diabetes. Studies using intravascular ultrasound have confirmed more extensive and more rapidly progressing CAD in diabetic subjects (Nicholls SJ et al., 2008).

Increased CVD risk also occurs with lesser degrees of dysglycaemia. For example, a systemic review by Ford ES et al. (2010) reported that both impaired fasting glucose and impaired glucose tolerance were associated with increased risk. Both 2-hour (Balkau B et al., 1998) and 1-hour (Orencia AJ et al., 1997) post-load glucose have associated with increased all-cause and CVD mortality in non-diabetic subjects. Similarly, 2-h post-load glucose ≥7.8 mmol/L was also reported to be predictive of the primary endpoint of CV mortality, nonfatal myocardial infarction, stroke, or hospitalization for heart failure in the EUROASPIRE survey (Shahim B et al., 2017). In a meta-analysis of 53 prospective cohort studies, Huang Y et al. (2016) found that both impaired glucose tolerance and impaired fasting glucose were associated with an increased risk of CVD, coronary heart disease, stroke, and all-cause mortality. In the same meta-analysis, increases in HBA_{1c} to 39-47 mmol/mol or 42-47 mmol/mol were both associated with an increased risk of CVD and coronary heart disease but not with an increased risk of stroke and all-cause mortality.

Another line of evidence to confirm the relation between high blood glucose and CVD is to investigate the effect of blood glucose lowering on CV disease and mortality. However, this has proven difficult to demonstrate in clinical trials. One reason may be due to the fact that it is difficult to lower blood glucose to the normal non-diabetic range at all times without risking hypoglycaemia.

The United Kingdom Prospective Study randomised newly diagnosed type 2 diabetic patients to standard or intensive glycaemic control for 10 years. There was a reduction in acute myocardial infarction by 16%, but this just failed to reach statistical significance (p = 0.052) (UK Prospective Diabetes Study (UKPDS) Group, 1998). However, epidemiological analysis of the UKPDS data, whereby patients were classified according to their mean HbA_{1c} irrespective of which arm they were allocated to, showed that there was a significant 14% reduction in MI for every 1% drop in mean HbA_{1c} (Stratton IM et al., 2000). The trialists of the UKPDS continued to collect data on the patients after study closure for a further 10 years. Even though mean HbA_{1c} was similar in the two groups during this observation period, the previously intensively treated group had a lower risk of MI and of death (Holman RR et al., 2008). This has introduced the concept of 'metabolic memory' or 'legacy effect', namely that tight glycaemic control early in the onset of the disease has long-term effects on complication risk.

Thereafter, subsequent studies similarly failed to show any benefit of intensive glycaemic control in type 2 diabetes on CV outcomes. These included the Action in Diabetes and Vascular Disease (ADVANCE) trial (ADVANCE Collaborative Group, 2008) and the Veterans Affairs Diabetes (VADT) Trial (Duckworth W et al., 2009). The Action to Control Cardiovascular Risk in Diabetes (ACCORD) Study had to be stopped prematurely because of increased mortality in the intensively treated arm (The ACCORD Study Group, 2008). The reason for the failure of these trials to show benefit of intensive glycaemic control may be related to their relatively short duration, small number of patients (VADT) and longer duration of diabetes and consequent metabolic memory of prior poor control. Another possibility is that the benefit of better glycaemic control might have been abrogated by the increased risk of hypoglycaemia associated with tighter glycaemic control. Hypoglycaemia is itself also associated with increased cardiovascular risk (Zoungas S et al., 2010; Lee AK et al., 2018). Similarly, the increased mortality observed in the ACCORD trial could be attributable to hypoglycaemia as a result of too aggressive blood glucose monitoring (Bonds DE et al., 2010).

More recently, use of sodium-glucose co-transporters inhibitors (Zinman B et al., 2015; Neal B et al., 2017; Wiviott SD et al., 2019) and some glucagon-like peptide analogues (Marso SP et al., 2016 (1); Marso SP et al., 2016 (2); Gerstein HC et al., 2019) have been shown to have significant cardiovascular benefit. It is unclear whether the beneficial effects of these novel agents are due to their propensity to lower blood glucose without hypoglycaemia or due to their pleiotropic, glucose-independent properties.

The mechanisms mediating the link between hyperglycaemia and vascular disease are complex, with many inter-linking pathways. These include hyperactivity of the polyol pathway (Dagher Z et al., 2004), generation of advanced glycation end-products (Goldin A et al., 2006; Yamagishi S et al., 2015), increased oxidative stress (Giacco F et al., 2010; Gray SP et al., 2013), and increased protein kinase C activity (Kizub IV et al., 2014; Tabit CE et al., 2013). There is also evidence of reduced endothelial progenitor cells (Saad MI et al., 2015). All these factors contribute to endothelial dysfunction and subclinical inflammation, both of which are commoner in diabetic subjects (Dhananjayan R et al., 2016; Li Q et al., 2012; Kampoli AM et al., 2011; Seligman BG et al., 2000; Makimattila S et al., 1996). Furthermore, diabetes is associated with a thrombophilic state. There is increased platelet activation (Véricel E et al., 2004) as well as abnormalities in both the coagulation and fibrinolytic pathways including hyperfibrinogenaemia (Sapkota B et al., 2013; Bembde AS et al., 2012) and increased plasminogen activator inhibitor-1 (Alzahrani SH et al., 2010). Increased protein glycation results in reduced plasmin generation from plasminogen (Ajjan RA et al., 2013) and resistance of fibrinogen to lysis (Pieters M et al., 2007).

DYSLIPIDAEMIA

There is a very strong link between high serum cholesterol and ischaemic heart disease in epidemiological studies. These include the Framingham Study (Kannel WB et al., 1971), the Multiple Risk Factor Intervention Trial [MRFIT] (Stamler J et al., 1993), the Chicago Heart Association Detection Project in Industry (Dyer AR et al., 1992), and the Peoples Gas Company Study (Dyer AR et al., 1975). Pooling of data from the last three-mentioned large cohorts showed a continuous, graded relationship of serum cholesterol level to long-term cardiovascular risk and all-cause mortality, and longer estimated life expectancy for younger men with favourable serum cholesterol levels (Stamler J et al., 2000). Numerous studies have confirmed that lowering cholesterol improves cardiovascular outcomes. These include the Scandinavian Simvastatin Survival Study (1994), the Long-Term Intervention with Pravastatin in Ischaemic Disease (LIPID) Study (1998) and the Anglo-Scandinavian Cardiac Outcomes Trial (Sever PS et al., 2003). Patients with the metabolic syndrome (Pyörälä K et al., 2004) or with diabetes (Colhoun HM et al., 2004; Cholesterol Treatment Trialists' (CTT) Collaborators, 2008) derive more benefit than the general population because of a higher background risk. Lowering serum cholesterol by non-statin drugs such as by proprotein convertase subtilisin/kexin type 9 inhibitors (Bonaca MP et al., 2018; AlTurki A et al., 2019) and ezetimibe (Cannon CP et al., 2015) has also been shown to reduce cardiovascular events. The fact that cholesterol lowering by different drugs having different modes of action is effective in reducing CVD strongly suggests that cholesterol is causally related to CVD. Higher intensity low-density lipoprotein (LDL) lowering is more effective in CVD reduction when compared to less intense lowering (Alkhalil M et al., 2020).

Lipids deposited in atheroma are derived from LDL and other apolipoprotein B (apo-B) containing lipoproteins. This explains the strong epidemiological association between LDL-cholesterol (LDL-C) and atherosclerotic disease (Wilson PW et al., 1998; Hargreaves AD et al., 1991; Sharrett AR et al., 2001). Furthermore LDL-C levels have been reported to correlate very strongly with coronary atherosclerosis progression as measured by intravascular ultrasound (Ray KK et al., 2007). Although LDL-C levels are normal in subjects with the metabolic syndrome or diabetes, they are still a very good indicator of risk (Gierach M et al., 2016; Turner RC et al., 1998).

In spite LDL-C levels being normal in insulin resistant states such as the metabolic syndrome, obesity and type 2 diabetes, there is more small dense LDL in these conditions (Austin MA et al., 1996; Sniderman AD et al., 2002; Garvey WT et al., 2003; Berneis K et al., 2005). Small dense LDL is more atherogenic as it is more likely to be oxidised and releases its cholesterol more readily (Tabas I, et al., 2007; Otvos JD et al., 2011; Wadhera RK et al., 2016). Insulin resistant states are associated with increased oxidised LDL (Trpkovic A et al., 2015). Oxidised LDL correlates with classical cardiovascular risk factors (Freitas MCP et al., 2018), but it also independently predicts 10-year progression of atherosclerosis as determined by carotid intima-media thickness (Gao S et al., 2018). A recent meta-analysis of 12 cohort studies (Gao S et al., 2017) found that oxidised LDL was associated with increased risk of atherosclerotic cardiovascular disease. Subsequently, oxidised LDL was reported to be associated with coronary artery disease (Zhang Q et al., 2019) and with prognosis after stroke (Wang A et al., 2017).

Insulin resistant states such as increased adiposity (both increased body mass index and increased waist circumference) are also associated with electronegatively charged LDL (LDL^{-ve}) (Freitas MCP et al., 2018; Hsu JF et al., 2014). Small particle size, glycosylation and non-esterified fatty acid enrichment (Akyol S et al., 2017) all predispose to the generation of LDL^{-ve} in insulin resistant states. LDL^{-ve} is highly atherogenic (Akyol S et al., 2017) through a number of mechanisms. These include its pro-inflammatory properties (Estruch M et al., 2013; Chu CS et al., 2013) and the induction of endothelial dysfunction (Lu J et al., 2008) and of endothelial senescence (Wang YC et al., 2018). It has also been reported to cause QT prolongation (Lee AS et al., 2017).

Apart from LDL-C, there are several other atherogenic lipid subfractions. These include the cholesterol-rich intermediate density lipoprotein, lipoprotein a [Lp(a)] and chylomicron remnants. Triglyceride-rich lipoproteins, such as chylomicrons and very-density lipoprotein also contribute to a lesser extent to the atherogenic part of total serum cholesterol. These subfractions are not measured in routine clinical practice, but the non-HDL cholesterol fraction captures cholesterol of all these atherogenic lipoprotein fractions (including LDL). For this reason, non-HDL cholesterol is a better indicator of cardiovascular risk than LDL-C (Cui Y et al., 2001; Wägner AM et al., 2003; Bittner V et al. 2005).

Apolipoprotein B (apo-B) is the principle apolipoprotein found in LDL and all the above-mentioned atherogenic lipoproteins, whilst the principle apolipoprotein of HDL is apolipoprotein A. There is one molecule of apo-B in every lipid particle, irrespective of its size. Apo-B therefore not only reflects total non-HDL cholesterol but also the number of atherogenic lipid particles. A high apo-B and a low LDL-C/apo-B ratio therefore predict the presence of small dense LDL (Wägner AM, et al., 2002; Wägner AM et al., 2003; Sniderman AD et al., 2019) and cardiovascular risk (Boekholdt SM et al., 2012).

Lp(a) is small particle bound to apoliporotein-a which has also been strongly linked to atherosclerotic disease (reviewed by Bucci M et al., 2016; Forbes CA et al., 2016). It has been shown to predict future cardiovascular events (Nicholls SJ et al., 2010; Nestel PJ et al., 2013; Emerging Risk Factors Collaboration, 2013). Genetically elevated Lp(a) is associated with increased risk of myocardial infarction (Kamstrup PR et al., 2009). Apart from being involved in lipid deposition, it is also pro-inflammatory and prothrombotic, promotes vascular smooth muscle proliferation, monocyte chemotaxis and foam cell formation (Ferretti G et al., 2018).

High-density lipoprotein (HDL) is important in transporting cholesterol away from cells, which referred to as reverse cholesterol transport. Additionally it has anti-oxidant properties and reduces oxidation of LDL (Van Lenten BJ et al., 1995); it also inhibits LDL-induced monocyte migration (Navab M et al., 1991). HDL-cholesterol (HDL-C) has been consistently shown to have an inverse relationship to cardiovascular risk in epidemiological studies (Wilson PW et al., 1988; Hargreaves AD et al., 1991; Assmann G et al., 1996; Wilson PW et al., 1998; Sharrett AR et al., 2001; Pischon T et al., 2005). In statin-treated patients HDL-C becomes the most important indicator of residual risk (Boekholdt SM et al., 2012; Boekholdt SM et al., 2013). Type 2 diabetic and other insulin resistant subjects have low HDL-C levels as a result of triglyceride enrichment which enhances their clearance by hepatic lipase (Després JP et al., 1989; Ginsberg HN et al., 2005). Reduced HDL in diabetic subjects correlates with increased risk (Turner RC et al., 1998). Insulin resistance is also associated with smaller HDL particles (Garvey WT et al., 2003), which has been linked to accelerated atherosclerosis (*Eckardstein A et al., 1994; Tomkin GH et al., 1994*). HDL particle number has been shown to be inversely associated with incident CVD (Khera AV et al., 2017). HDL contains apolipoprotein-A (apo-A), whilst atherogenic lipoproteins contain apolipoprotein-B (apo-B). For this reason, the apo-B/apo-A ratio was found to be a strong predictor of acute myocardial infarction in the INTERHEART (Yusuf S et al., 2004; McQueen MJ et al., 2008) and AMORIS (Walldius G et al., 2001; Holme I et al., 2008) studies.

In subjects with type 2 diabetes, not only is HDL reduced, but is also dysfunctional as a result of oxidative modification and glycation of the HDL protein (Srivastava RAK, 2018; Femlak M et al., 2017; Vaisar T et al., 2018). This affects both its reverse cholesterol and anti-oxidative properties. Such dysfunctional HDL is associated with a greater risk of CVD (Soria-Florido MT et al., 2020).

Finally hypertriglyceridaemia has also been associated with cardiovascular risk (Castelli WP et al., 1992; Eberly LE et al., 2003; de

Jongh RT et al., 2004; Nordestgaard BG et al., 2007; Sarwar N et al., 2007). Insulin decreases very low density lipoprotein production by the liver (Lewis GF et al., 1993) and stimulates lipoprotein lipase thereby accelerating clearing of plasma triglycerides (Taskinen MR et al., 1982). This explains the increase in serum triglycerides observed in insulin resistant states (Ginsberg HN et al., 2005). Hypertriglyceridaemia results in triglyceride enrichment of HDL accelerating its clearance as described above. The increased CV risk associated with hypertriglyceridaemia may therefore be driven by its HDL-lowering effects. Other potential mechanisms including the association of hypertriglyceridaemia with obesity, insulin resistance and elevated circulating free fatty acids (FFA). The latter have been reported to cause endothelial dysfunction (Newens KJ et al., 2015; Steinberg HO et al., 1997; Steinberg HO et al., 2000; Perassolo MS et al. 2008) and to be associated with hypertension (Fagot-Campagna A et al., 1998). FFA have also been reported to adversely affect myocardial function and cause myocardial insulin resistance in rats (Han L et al., 2018) as well as cause endothelial progenitor cell senescence (Song X et al., 2017). Furthermore, they have been shown to be associated with arterial stiffness in the general population (Tabara Y et al., 2016). In the Québec Cardiovascular Study, elevated plasma FFA concentrations were associated with an increased risk of ischaemic heart disease (Pirro M et al., 2002), whilst Pilz S et al. (2006) found that elevated circulating free fatty acids were associated with increased all-cause and cardiovascular mortality in subjects with coronary artery disease. Very recently reduction of serum triglycerides by icosapent ethyl has been reported to reduce cardiovascular risk (Bhatt DL et al., 2019).

HYPERTENSION

Although hypertension is strictly speaking not a metabolic condition, it is one of the criteria used in the definition of the metabolic syndrome and of metabolic health (see below). It has long been established as one of the risk factors for cardiovascular events identified in several key epidemiological studies, including the Framingham study (Kannel WB et al., 1972; Kannel WB et al., 1975), the MRFIT study (Stamler J et al., 1989; Flack JM et al., 1995), the Chicago Heart Association Detection Project in Industry (Miura K et al., 2001), the INTERHEART study (Yusuf S et al., 2004; Lanas F et al., 2007), the Avoiding Cardiovascular events through Combination therapy in Patients Living with Systolic Hypertension (ACCOMPLISH) trial (Weber MA et al., 2007) and others (e.g., McCarron et al., 2000; Yano Y et al., 2020). Hypertension is a CV risk factor even in elderly subjects (Vokonas PS et al., 1988). Isolated systolic hypertension is also associated with increased risk of both coronary heart disease and cardiovascular disease mortality as demonstrated by Yano Y et al. (2015).

The mechanisms mediating the increased risk associated with hypertension include endothelial injury as a result of mechanical stress causing endothelial dysfunction (*Panza JA* et al., 1990; *Linder L* et al., 1990; *Panza JA* et al., 1993). Hypertension also results in increased after-load and left ventricular hypertrophy, which is known to be associated with cardiovascular disease. Furthermore hypertension, as part of the metabolic syndrome is commonly associated with insulin resistance, dysglycaemia and increased adiposity.

There were several trials comparing antihypertensive treatment with placebo. These are reviewed in the National Institute of Health and Clinical Excellence guidelines (NICE, 2019). Intensive blood pressure control has been reported to reduce cardiovascular events in patients both with and without diabetes (SPRINT Research Group et al., 2015; Brouwer TF et al., 2018). There is also evidence for a legacy effect of blood pressure medications (Gupta A et al., 2018).

ADIPOSITY

Obesity is another well-established risk factor for cardiovascular disease. For example, the Framingham study found that the percentage of desirable weight at baseline predicted 26-year incidence of coronary disease, coronary death and congestive heart failure in men independently of age, cholesterol, systolic blood pressure, smoking, left ventricular hypertrophy and glucose intolerance (Hubert HB et al., 1983). Weight gain was associated with an increased risk of CVD in both sexes. The Chicago Heart Association Detection Project in Industry study had similar results with obesity being associated with increased 25-year cardiovascular risk (Dyer AR et al., 2004). Similarly Jousilahti P et al. (1996) found that body mass index (BMI) was associated with increased coronary heart disease mortality in a large prospective study of subjects aged 30 to 59 years. In the case-control INTERHEART study BMI had graded association with myocardial infarction (Yusuf S et al., 2005). There is also a strong link of obesity with increased mortality (Berrington de Gonzalez A et al., 2010; Masters RK et al., 2013).

Various studies have now demonstrated that central obesity is more strongly associated with cardiovascular risk (Rexrode KM et al., 1998; Dagenais GR et al., 2005; Yusuf S et al., 2005) as well as with cardiovascular and all-cause mortality (Lim RB et al., 2015) than BMI; and this relationship occurs across all categories of BMI. Central obesity is also a stronger predictor of diabetes than BMI (Li C et al., 2010). Because obesity is increasing worldwide at an alarming rate (World Health Organization, 2000), the population attributable risk of cardiovascular disease associated with obesity is substantial and is likely to continue to increase.

The association of increased adiposity to cardiovascular disease is probably mediated through its association with insulin resistance/hyperinsulinaemia, increased circulating free fatty acids, and an unfavourable adipokine profile. The latter includes high tumour-necrosis factor-α and interleukin-6 and reduced adiponectin (Kougias P et al., 2005; Bahceci M et al., 2007; Lau DC et al., 2015; Blüher M et al., 2016; Fasshauer M & Blüher M, 2015; Park HK et al., 2017). All these factors predispose to subclinical inflammation (Xu H et al., 2003; Bastard JP et al., 2006; Garanty-Bogacka B et al., 2005) and endothelial dysfunction (Garanty-Bogacka B et al., 2005), which are known to be common in obese subjects (Pontiroli AE et al., 2004). High circulating FFA, resistin and TNF-α also predispose to insulin resistance. In obese individuals, there is also increased small dense LDL (Kang HS et al., 2002), which, as discussed above is highly atherogenic. Obesity is also associated with pancreatic islet inflammation which impairs pancreatic β-cell-function. There is also β-cell lipotoxicity from high circulating triglycerides and FFA (Song Z et al., 2019), further predisposing to diabetes (Ying W et al., 2020).

CLUSTERING OF METABOLIC ABNORMALITIES

The interrelationships of cardiometabolic abnormalities described above are summarised in Figure 1. Because of these interrelationships, cardiometabolic abnormalities tend to cluster in the same individual. The most widely accepted term to capture this clustering of adverse metabolic abnormalities is that of the metabolic syndrome. Unfortunately, there are different definitions to this term so that there is heterogeneity to what authors refer to in the literature. The most commonly used definitions are those of the International Diabetes Federation (Alberti KG et al., 2005), the World Health Organisation (2009) and the National Cholesterol Education Program (NCEP) III (2002). These are summarised in Table 1. Although the validity of the concept of the metabolic syndrome has been questioned (Kahn R et al., 2005), it has been shown in large studies to predict cardiovascular disease irrespective of the definition used (De Simone G et al., 2007; Lorenzo C et al., 2007; Dekker JM et al., 2005; Pajunen P et al., 2010; Lakka HM et al., 2002). This also holds true in diabetic subjects (De Simone G et al., 2007; Bonora E et al., 2004). A meta-analysis by Gami et al. (2007) found that the metabolic syndrome was associated with increased cardiovascular risk even after adjusting for traditional risk factors, with the strongest association being observed with the WHO definition. A consensus definition of the metabolic syndrome has also been proposed (Alberti KG et al., 2009). This requires any 3 of high waist circumference, high serum triglycerides, low HDL-C, high systolic or diastolic blood pressure and high blood glucose or use of anti-hyperglycaemic control. Importantly, the metabolic syndrome as determined by this consensus definition was shown to be a better predictor of incident CVD than the sum of its components in the Health 2000 study (Pajunen P et al., 2010). It was also a better predictor of CVD than the Framingham risk score in women, but not in men. Similarly, Wannamethee SG et al. (2005) had shown that the Framingham risk score was a better predictor of coronary heart disease in middle-aged men.

Table 1. Definitions of the metabolic syndrome as proposed by different organisations

Clinical parameter	World Health Organisation (WHO), 1999	National Cholesterol Education Program (NCEP) Expert Panel on Detection, Evaluation and Treatment of High blood Cholesterol in Adults (ATPIIII), 2001	International Diabetes Federation (IDF), 2006
Insulin Resistance	High insulin levels, IGT, IFG or T2 DM Plus, any two of the following:	None, but Any three of the following:	None
Abdominal obesity:	WHR >0.9 in males or >0.85 in women; and/or BMI > 30kg/m^2,	WC >102cm for men and >88cm for women	Central obesity as defined by ethnic/racial specific WC and two of the following:
Blood Pressure	>140/90 mmHg	>130/85 mmHg	>130/85 or on treatment
Lipid Profile	TG > 1.7mmol/l or HDL-C < 0.9 mmol/l in men and <1.0 mmol/l in women	TG > 1.7 mmol/l HDL-C: <1.03 mmol/l for men and <1.3 mmol/l for women	TG >1.7 mmol/l or on treatment HDL-C: <1.03 mmol/l for men, <1.3 mmol/l for women or on treatment
Glucose	IGT, IFG or T2 DM	FPG > 5.6 mmol/l	FPG >5.6 mmol/l
Other Criteria	Microalbuminuria: ACR >30mg/g		

IGT: impaired glucose tolerance, IFG: impaired fasting glucose, T2 DM: type 2 diabetes, TG: triglycerides, HDL-C: high-density cholesterol, FPG: fasting plasma glucose, ACR: albumin : creatinine ratio.

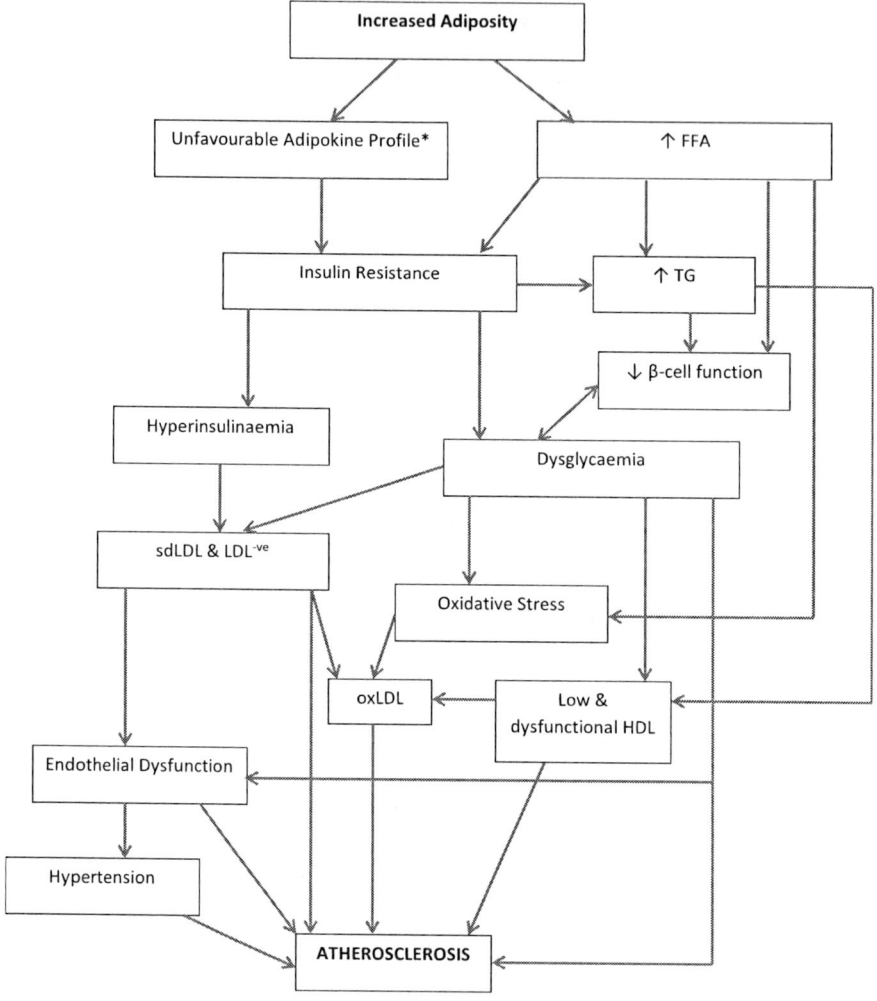

Figure 1. Summary of the interrelations of metabolic abnormalities and pathways leading to atherosclerosis. Many of these cardiometabolic abnormalities also predispose to a thrombophilic state and to myocardial injury. See text for further detail. FFA = free fatty acids; HDL = high density lipoprotein; LDL^{-ve} = electronegatively charged low-density lipoprotein; oxLDL = oxidised low-density lipoprotein; sdLDL = small dense low-density lipoprotein; TG = triglycerides. * refers to low adiponection, high inteleukin-6 & high resistin levels.

A relatively newer way to describe clustering of metabolic factors associated with cardiovascular risk is the concept of metabolic health. Unfortunately, there is no universally accepted definition of what constitutes metabolic health. All definitions use different combinations of the cardiometabolic abnormalities described above including insulin resistance, high serum triglycerides, low HDL-C, high blood pressure and dysglycaemia. They vary in how insulin resistance is defined, in cut-offs used and in how many abnormal parameters are needed to define the metabolic unhealthy state. Methods used by authors to measure insulin resistance include the hyperinsulinaemic-euglycemic clamp, insulin sensitivity after an oral glucose tolerance test and the homeostatic model assessment of insulin resistance (HOMA-IR). The National Health and Nutrition Examination Surveys (NHANES) study of the United States defined metabolic healthiness as having one or no cardiometabolic abnormalities, whereas metabolic unhealthiness was defined as the presence of two or more of such abnormalities (Wildman et al., 2008). The metabolic abnormalities included elevated blood pressure; elevated levels of triglycerides, fasting plasma glucose, and C-reactive protein; elevated homeostasis model assessment of insulin resistance value; and low high-density lipoprotein cholesterol level. On the other hand most other studies did not include insulin resistance or subclinical inflammation and used the presence of fewer than two parameters of the metabolic syndrome to full fill the criteria of metabolic healthiness (Kramer et al., 2013; Stefan et al., 2013).

Although obesity is strongly associated with an adverse cardiometabolic profile, there are some overweight or obese individuals who are metabolically healthy. These are referred to as metabolically healthy obese individuals to distinguish them from the commoner metabolically unhealthy obese. Similarly, there are also some normal weight individuals who are metabolically unhealthy and are at higher cardiovascular risk (Brant LC et al., 2017). These are referred to as metabolically unhealthy normal weight individuals to distinguish them from the commoner metabolically healthy normal weight individuals (reviewed by Fava MC et al., 2019). Metabolically healthy obese may be have a cardiovascular risk which is intermediate between that of metabolically healthy normal weight and metabolically unhealthy obese individuals (Eckel N et al. 2016).

CONCLUSION

A large array of inter-related metabolic abnormalities is of central importance in the pathogenesis of cardiovascular disease. These abnormalities include hyperinsulinaemia, insulin resistance, low and dysfunctional HDL, modified LDL (small dense LDL, oxidised LDL, electronegatively charged LDL), hypertriglyceridaemia, high circulating free fatty acids and dysglycaemia. These lead to oxidative stress, subclinical inflammation, endothelial dysfunction, accelerated atherogenesis and thrombophilia. Amelioration of many of these factors has been shown to improve cardiovascular outcomes. The concept of the metabolic syndrome and that of metabolic unhealthiness attempt to capture clustering of these metabolic abnormalities in the same individual. Adiposity is strongly linked with the metabolic syndrome, absence of metabolic health and with many of the individual metabolic abnormalities.

REFERENCES

Action to Control Cardiovascular Risk in Diabetes Study Group, Gerstein HC, Miller ME, Byington RP, Goff DC Jr, Bigger JT, Buse JB, Cushman WC, Genuth S, Ismail-Beigi F, Grimm RH Jr, Probstfield JL, Simons-Morton DG, Friedewald WT. Effects of intensive glucose lowering in type 2 diabetes. *N Engl J Med* 2008;358:2545-59.

ADVANCE Collaborative Group, Patel A, MacMahon S, Chalmers J, Neal B, Billot L, Woodward M, Marre M, Cooper M, Glasziou P, Grobbee D, Hamet P, Harrap S, Heller S, Liu L, Mancia G, Mogensen CE, Pan C, Poulter N, Rodgers A, Williams B, Bompoint S, de Galan BE, Joshi R, Travert F. Intensive blood glucose control and vascular outcomes in patients with type 2 diabetes. *N Engl J Med.* 2008;358:2560-72.

Ajjan RA, Gamlen T, Standeven KF, Mughal S, Hess K, Smith KA, Dunn EJ, Anwar MM, Rabbani N, Thornalley PJ, Philippou H, Grant PJ. Diabetes is associated with posttranslational modifications in plasminogen resulting in reduced plasmin generation and enzyme-specific activity. *Blood.* 2013;122:134-42.

Akyol S, Lu J, Akyol O, Akcay F, Armutcu F, Ke LY, Chen CH. The role of electronegative low-density lipoprotein in cardiovascular diseases and its therapeutic implications. *Trends Cardiovasc Med.* 2017;27:239-246.

Alberti KG, Eckel RH, Grundy SM, Zimmet PZ, Cleeman JI, Donato KA, Fruchart JC, James WP, Loria CM, Smith SC Jr; International Diabetes Federation Task Force on Epidemiology and Prevention; Hational Heart, Lung, and Blood Institute; American Heart Association; World Heart Federation; International Atherosclerosis Society; International Association for the Study of Obesity. Harmonizing the metabolic syndrome: a joint interim statement of the International Diabetes Federation Task Force on Epidemiology and Prevention; National Heart, Lung, and Blood Institute; American Heart Association; World Heart Federation; International Atherosclerosis Society; and International Association for the Study of Obesity. *Circulation.* 2009;120:1640-5.

Alberti KG, Zimmet P, Shaw J, The IDF Epidemiology Task Force Consensus Group: The metabolic syndrome: a new worldwide definition. *Lancet.* 366:1059-1062, 2005.

Alkhalil M. Effects of intensive lipid-lowering therapy on mortality after coronary bypass surgery: A meta-analysis of 7 randomised trials. *Atherosclerosis.* 2020;293:75-78.

AlTurki A, Marafi M, Dawas A, Dube MP, Vieira L, Sherman MH, Gregoire J, Alzahrani SH, Ajjan RA. Coagulation and fibrinolysis in diabetes. *Diab Vasc Dis Res.* 2010;7:260-273.

Assmann G, Schulte H, von Eckardstein A, Huang Y. High-density lipoprotein cholesterol as a predictor of coronary heart disease risk. The PROCAM experience and pathophysiological implications for reverse cholesterol transport. *Atherosclerosis.* 1996;124 Suppl:S11-20.

Bahceci M, Gokalp D, Bahceci S, Tuzcu A, Atmaca S, Arikan S. The correlation between adiposity and adiponectin, tumor necrosis factor a, interleukin-6 and high sensitivity C-reactive protein levels. Is adipocyte size associated with inflammation in adults? *J. Endocrinol. Invest.* 2007; 30, 210-214.

Balbay Y, Gagnon-Arpin I, Malhan S, Öksüz ME, Sutherland G, Dobrescu A, Villa G, Ertuğrul G, Habib M. Modeling the burden of cardiovascular disease in Turkey. *Anatol J Cardiol.* 2018;20:235-240.

Balkau B, Shipley M, Jarrett RJ, Pyörälä K, Pyörälä M, Forhan A, Eschwège E. High blood glucose concentration is a risk factor for mortality in middle-aged nondiabetic men. 20-year follow-up in the Whitehall Study, the Paris Prospective Study, and the Helsinki Policemen Study. *Diabetes Care.* 1998;21:360-7.

Bastard JP, Maachi M, Lagathu C et al. Recent advances in the relationship between obesity, inflammation, and insulin resistance. *Eur. Cytokine Netw.* 2006;17, 4-12.

Bembde AS. A study of plasma fibrinogen level in type-2 diabetes mellitus and its relation to glycemic control. *Indian J Hematol Blood Transfus.* 2012;28:105-8.

Berrington de Gonzalez A, Hartge P, Cerhan JR, Flint AJ, Hannan L, MacInnis RJ, Moore SC, Tobias GS, Anton-Culver H, Freeman LB, Beeson WL, Clipp SL, English DR, Folsom AR, Freedman DM, Giles G, Hakansson N, Henderson KD, Hoffman-Bolton J, Hoppin JA, Koenig KL, Lee IM, Linet MS, Park Y, Pocobelli G, Schatzkin A, Sesso HD, Weiderpass E, Willcox BJ, Wolk A, Zeleniuch-Jacquotte A, Willett WC, Thun MJ. Body-mass index and mortality among 1.46 million white adults. *N Engl J Med.* 2010;363:2211-9.

Bhatt DL, Steg PG, Miller M, Brinton EA, Jacobson TA, Ketchum SB, Doyle RT Jr,Juliano RA, Jiao L, Granowitz C, Tardif JC, Ballantyne CM; REDUCE-IT Investigators. Cardiovascular Risk Reduction with Icosapent Ethyl for Hypertriglyceridemia. *N Engl J Med.* 2019;380:11-22.

Blüher M. Adipose tissue inflammation: a cause or consequence of obesity-related insulin resistance? *Clin Sci (Lond).* 2016;130:1603-14.

Boekholdt SM, Arsenault BJ, Hovingh GK, et al. Levels and changes of HDL cholesterol and apolipoprotein A-I in relation to risk of cardiovascular events among statin-treated patients: a meta-analysis. *Circulation.* 2013;128:1504–1512.

Boekholdt SM, Arsenault BJ, Mora S, et al. Association of LDL cholesterol, non-HDL cholesterol, and apolipoprotein B levels with risk of cardiovascular events among patients treated with statins: a meta-analysis. *JAMA.* 2012;307:1302–1309.

Bonaca MP, Nault P, Giugliano RP, Keech AC, Pineda AL, Kanevsky E, Kuder J, Murphy SA, Jukema JW, Lewis BS, Tokgozoglu L, Somaratne R, Sever PS, Pedersen TR, Sabatine MS. Low-Density Lipoprotein Cholesterol Lowering With Evolocumab and Outcomes in Patients With Peripheral Artery Disease: Insights From the FOURIER Trial (Further Cardiovascular Outcomes Research With PCSK9 Inhibition in Subjects With Elevated Risk). *Circulation.* 2018;137:338-350.

Bonds DE, Miller ME, Bergenstal RM, Buse JB, Byington RP, Cutler JA, Dudl RJ, Ismail-Beigi F, Kimel AR, Hoogwerf B, Horowitz KR, Savage PJ, Seaquist ER, Simmons DL, Sivitz WI, Speril-Hillen JM, Sweeney ME. The association between symptomatic, severe hypoglycaemia and mortality in type 2 diabetes: retrospective epidemiological analysis of the ACCORD study. *BMJ.* 2010; 340:b4909.

Bonora E, Targher G, Formentini G, Calcaterra F, Lombardi S, Marini F, Zenari L, Saggiani F, Poli M, Perbellini S, Raffaelli A, Gemma L, Santi L, Bonadonna RC, Muggeo M: The metabolic syndrome is an independent predictor of cardiovascular disease in type 2 diabetic subjects: prospective data from the Verona Diabetes Complications Study. *Diabet Med.* 2004; 21:52-584.

Brant LC, Wang N, Ojeda FM, LaValley M, Barreto SM, Benjamin EJ, Mitchell GF, Vasan RS, Palmisano JN, Münzel T, Blankenberg S, Wild PS, Zeller T, Ribeiro AL, Schnabel RB, Hamburg NM. Relations of Metabolically Healthy and Unhealthy Obesity to Digital Vascular Function in Three Community-Based Cohorts: A Meta-Analysis. *J Am Heart Assoc.* 2017;6(3) pii: e004199.

Brouwer TF, Vehmeijer JT, Kalkman DN, Berger WR, van den Born BH, Peters RJ, Knops RE. Intensive Blood Pressure Lowering in Patients

With and Patients Without Type 2 Diabetes: A Pooled Analysis From Two Randomized Trials. *Diabetes Care.* 2018;41:1142-1148.

Bucci M, Tana C, Giamberardino MA, Cipollone F. Lp(a) and cardiovascular risk: Investigating the hidden side of the moon. *Nutr Metab Cardiovasc Dis.* 2016. pii: S0939-4753(16)30111-9.

Cannon CP, Blazing MA, Giugliano RP, McCagg A, White JA, Theroux P, Darius H, Lewis BS, Ophuis TO, Jukema JW, De Ferrari GM, Ruzyllo W, De Lucca P, Im K, Bohula EA, Reist C, Wiviott SD, Tershakovec AM, Musliner TA, Braunwald E, Califf RM; IMPROVE-IT Investigators. Ezetimibe Added to Statin Therapy after Acute Coronary Syndromes. *N Engl J Med.* 2015;372:2387-97.

Castelli WP. Epidemiology of triglycerides: a view from Framingham. *Am J Cardiol.* 1992;70:3H-9H.

Cholesterol Treatment Trialists' (CTT) Collaborators, Kearney PM, Blackwell L, Collins R, Keech A, Simes J, Peto R, Armitage J, Baigent C. Efficacy of cholesterol-lowering therapy in 18,686 people with diabetes in 14 randomised trials of statins: a meta-analysis. *Lancet.* 2008;371(9607):117-25.

Chu CS, Wang YC, Lu LS, et al. Electronegative low-density lipoprotein increases C-reactive protein expression in vascular endothelial cells through the LOX-1 receptor. *PLoS One.* 2013;8(8):e70533.

Colhoun HM, Betteridge DJ, Durrington PN, Hitman GA, Neil HA, Livingstone SJ, homason MJ, Mackness MI, Charlton-Menys V, Fuller JH; CARDS investigators. Primary prevention of cardiovascular disease with atorvastatin in type 2 diabetes in the Collaborative Atorvastatin Diabetes Study (CARDS): multicentre randomised placebo-controlled trial. *Lancet.* 2004;364:685-96.

Cui Y, Blumenthal RS, Flaws JA, Whiteman MK, Langenberg P, Bachorik PS, Bush TL: Non-high-density lipoprotein cholesterol level as a predictor of cardiovascular disease mortality. *Arch Intern Med.* 2001; 161:1413–1419.

Dagenais GR, Yi Q, Mann JF, Bosch J, Pogue J, Yusuf S. Prognostic impact of body weight and abdominal obesity in women and men with cardiovascular disease. *Am Heart J.* 2005;149:54-60.

Dagher Z, Park YS, Asnaghi V, Hoehn T, Gerhardinger C, Lorenzi M. Studies of rat and human retinas predict a role for the polyol pathway in human diabetic retinopathy. *Diabetes.* 2004;53:2404-11.

de Jongh RT, Serne EH, Ijzerman RG, de Vries G, Stehouwer CD. Free fatty acid levels modulate microvascular function: relevance for obesity-associated insulin resistance, hypertension, and microangiopathy. *Diabetes.* 2004; 53, 2873-2882.

De Simone G, Devereux RB, Chinali M. Strong Heart Study Investigators Prognostic impact of metabolic syndrome by different definitions in a population with high prevalence of obesity and diabetes: the Strong Heart Study. *Diabetes Care.* 2007; 30: 1851–1856.

Dekker JM, Girman C, Rhodes T. Metabolic syndrome and 10-year cardiovascular disease risk in the Hoorn Study. *Circulation.* 2005; 112: 666–673.

Després JP, Ferland M, Moorjani S, Nadeau A, Tremblay A, Lupien PJ, Thériault G, Bouchard C. Role of hepatic-triglyceride lipase activity in the association between intra-abdominal fat and plasma HDL cholesterol in obese women. *Arteriosclerosis.* 1989;9:485-92.

Dhananjayan R, Koundinya KS, Malati T, Kutala VK. Endothelial Dysfunction in Type 2 Diabetes Mellitus. *Indian J Clin Biochem.* 2016;31:372-9.

Duckworth W, Abraira C, Moritz T, Reda D, Emanuele N, Reaven PD, Zieve FJ, Marks J, Davis SN, Hayward R, Warren SR, Goldman S, McCarren M, Vitek ME, Henderson WG, Huang GD; VADT Investigators. Glucose control and vascular complications in veterans with type 2 diabetes. *N Engl J Med.* 2009;360:129-39.

Dyer AR, Stamler J, Garside DB, Greenland P. Long-term consequences of body mass index for cardiovascular mortality: the Chicago Heart Association Detection Project in Industry study. *Ann Epidemiol.* 2004;14:101-8.

Eberly LE, Stamler J, Neaton JD; Multiple Risk Factor Intervention Trial Research Group. Relation of triglyceride levels, fasting and nonfasting, to fatal and nonfatal coronary heart disease. *Arch Intern Med.* 2003;163:1077-83.

Eckardstein A, Huang Y, Assmann G. Physiological role and clinical relevance of high-density lipoprotein subclasses. *Curr Opin Lipidol* 5: 404 –416,1994.

Eckel N, Meidtner K, Kalle-Uhlmann T, Stefan N, Schulze MB (2016). Metabolically healthy obesity and cardiovascular events: a systematic review and meta-analysis. *Eur J Prev Cardiol* 23:956–966.

Emerging Risk Factors Collaboration, Erqou S, Kaptoge S, Perry PL, Di Angelantonio E, Thompson A, White IR, Marcovina SM, Collins R, Thompson SG, Danesh J. Lipoprotein(a) concentration and the risk of coronary heart disease, stroke, and nonvascular mortality. *JAMA.* 2009;302:412-23.

Estruch M, Sánchez-Quesada JL, Ordóñez Llanos J, Benítez S. Electronegative LDL: a circulating modified LDL with a role in inflammation. *Mediators Inflamm.* 2013; 2013:181324.

Fagot-Campagna A, Balkau B, Simon D et al. High free fatty acid concentration: an independent risk factor for hypertension in the Paris Prospective Study. *Int J Epidemiol.* 1998; 27, 808-813.

Falcao-Pires I, Leite-Moreira AF. Diabetic cardiomyopathy: understanding the molecular and cellular basis to progress in diagnosis and treatment. *Heart Fail. Rev.* 2012;17:325–344.

Fasshauer M, Blüher M. Adipokines in health and disease. *Trends Pharmacol Sci.* 2015;36:461-70.

Fava MC, Agius R, Fava S. Obesity and cardio-metabolic health. *Br J Hosp Med* (Lond). 2019;80:466-471.

Femlak M, Gluba-Brzózka A, Ciałkowska-Rysz A, Rysz J. The role and function of HDL in patients with diabetes mellitus and the related cardiovascular risk. *Lipids Health Dis.* 2017;16:207.

Ferretti G, Bacchetti T, Johnston TP, Banach M, Pirro M, Sahebkar A. Lipoprotein(a): A missing culprit in the management of athero-thrombosis? *J Cell Physiol.* 2018;233:2966-2981.

Flack JM, Neaton J, Grimm R Jr, Shih J, Cutler J, Ensrud K, MacMahon S. Blood pressure and mortality among men with prior myocardial infarction. Multiple Risk Factor Intervention Trial Research Group. *Circulation.* 1995;92:2437-45.

Fontbonne AM, Eschwège EM. Insulin and cardiovascular disease. Paris Prospective Study. *Diabetes Care.* 1991;14:461-9.

Forbes CA, Quek RG, Deshpande S, Worthy G, Wolff R, Stirk L, Kleijnen J, Gandra SR, Djedjos S, Wong ND. The relationship between Lp(a) and CVD outcomes: a systematic review. *Lipids Health Dis.* 2016;15:95.

Ford ES, Zhao G, Li C. Pre-diabetes and the risk for cardiovascular disease: a systematic review of the evidence. *J Am Coll Cardiol.* 2010;55:1310-7.

Freitas MCP, Fernandez DGE, Cohen D, Figueiredo-Neto AM, Maranhão RC, Damasceno NRT. Oxidized and electronegative low-density lipoprotein as potential biomarkers of cardiovascular risk in obese adolescents. *Clinics (Sao Paulo).* 2018;73:e189.

Gami AS, Witt BJ, Howard DE, Erwin PJ, Gami LA, Somers VK, Montori VM. Metabolic syndrome and risk of incident cardiovascular events and death: asystematic review and meta-analysis of longitudinal studies. *J Am Coll Cardiol* 2007;49:403-14.

Gao S, Zhao D, Qi Y, Wang W, Wang M, Sun J, Liu J, Li Y, Liu J. Circulating Oxidized Low-Density Lipoprotein Levels Independently Predict 10-Year Progression of Subclinical Carotid Atherosclerosis: A Community-Based Cohort Study. *J Atheroscler Thromb.* 2018;25:1032-1043.

Gao S, Zhao D, Wang M, Zhao F, Han X, Qi Y, Liu J. Association Between Circulating Oxidized LDL and Atherosclerotic Cardiovascular Disease: A Meta-analysis of Observational Studies. *Can J Cardiol.* 2017; 33:1624-1632.

Garanty-Bogacka B, Syrenicz M, Syrenicz A, Gebala A, Lulka D, Walczak M. Serum markers of inflammation and endothelial activation in children with obesity-related hypertension. *Neuro. Endocrinol. Lett.* 2005; 26, 242-246.

Garvey WT, Kwon S, Zheng D, Shaughnessy S, Wallace P, Hutto A, Pugh K, Jenkins AJ, Klein RL, Liao Y. Effects of insulin resistance and type 2 diabetes on lipoprotein subclass particle size and concentration determined by nuclear magnetic resonance. *Diabetes.* 2003;52:453-62.

Gerstein HC, Colhoun HM, Dagenais GR, Diaz R, Lakshmanan M, Pais P,Probstfield J, Riesmeyer JS, Riddle MC, Rydén L, Xavier D, Atisso CM, Dyal L,Hall S, Rao-Melacini P, Wong G, Avezum A, Basile J, Chung N, Conget I, Cushman WC, Franek E, Hancu N, Hanefeld M, Holt S, Jansky P, Keltai M, Lanas F, Leiter LA, Lopez-Jaramillo P, Cardona Munoz EG, Pirags V, Pogosova N, Raubenheimer PJ,Shaw JE, Sheu WH, Temelkova-Kurktschiev T; REWIND Investigators. Dulaglutide and cardiovascular outcomes in type 2 diabetes (REWIND): a double-blind, randomised placebo-controlled trial. *Lancet.* 2019; 394(10193):121-130.

Giacco F, Brownlee M. Oxidative stress and diabetic complications. *Circ Res.* 2010;107:1058-70.

Gierach M, Gierach J, Junik R. Evaluation of lipid profiles in patients with metabolic syndrome according to cardiovascular risk calculated on the basis of the SCORE chart. *Endokrynol Pol.* 2016;67:265-70.

Ginsberg HN, Zhang YL, Hernandez-Ono A. Regulation of plasma triglycerides in insulin resistance and diabetes. *Arch Med Res.* 2005;36:232-40.

Goldin A, Beckman JA, Schmidt AM, Creager MA. Advanced glycation end products: sparking the development of diabetic vascular injury. *Circulation.* 2006;114:597–605.

Gray SP, Di Marco E, Okabe J, Szyndralewiez C, Heitz F, Montezano AC, de Haan JB, Koulis C, El-Osta A, Andrews KL, Chin-Dusting JP, Touyz RM, Wingler K, Cooper ME, Schmidt HH, Jandeleit-Dahm KA. NADPH oxidase 1 plays a key role in diabetes mellitus-accelerated atherosclerosis. *Circulation* 2013;127:1888-902.

Gupta A, Mackay J, Whitehouse A, Godec T, Collier T, Pocock S, Poulter N, Sever P. Long-term mortality after blood pressure-lowering and lipid-lowering treatment in patients with hypertension in the Anglo-Scandinavian Cardiac Outcomes Trial (ASCOT) Legacy study: 16-year follow-up results of a randomised factorial trial. *Lancet.* 2018 Sep 29;392(10153):1127-1137.

Gupta A, Mackay J, Whitehouse A, Godec T, Collier T, Pocock S, Poulter N, Sever P. Long-term mortality after blood pressure-lowering and lipid-lowering treatment in patients with hypertension in the Anglo-Scandinavian Cardiac Outcomes Trial (ASCOT) Legacy study: 16-year follow-up results of a randomised factorial trial. *Lancet.* 2018; 392(10153):1127-1137.

Han L, Liu J, Zhu L, Tan F, Qin Y, Huang H, Yu Y. Free fatty acid can induce cardiac dysfunction and alter insulin signaling pathways in the heart. *Lipids Health Dis.* 2018;17:185.

Hargreaves AD, Logan RL, Thomson M, Elton RA, Oliver MF, Riemersma RA. Total cholesterol, low density lipoprotein cholesterol, and high density lipoprotein cholesterol and coronary heart disease in Scotland. *BMJ.* 1991;303(6804):678-81.

Holman RR, Paul SK, Bethel MA, Matthews DR, Neil HA. 10-year follow-up of intensive glucose control in type 2 diabetes. *N Engl J Med* 2008;359:1577-89.

Holme I, Aastveit AH, Jungner I, Walldius G. Relationships between lipoprotein components and risk of myocardial infarction: age, gender and short versus longer follow-up periods in the Apolipoprotein MOrtality RISk study (AMORIS). *J Intern Med.* 2008;264:30-8.

Hsu JF, Chou TC, Lu J, Chen SH, Chen FY, Chen CC, Chen JL, Elayda M, Ballantyne CM, Shayani S, Chen CH. Low-density lipoprotein electronegativity is a novel cardiometabolic risk factor. *PLoS One.* 2014;9(9):e107340.

Hu G, Qiao Q, Tuomilehto J, Eliasson M, Feskens EJ, Pyörälä K, The DECODE Insulin Study Group. Plasma insulin and cardiovascular mortality in non-diabetic European men and women: a meta-analysis of data from eleven prospective studies. *Diabetologia.* 2004; 47, 1245-1256.

Huang Y, Cai X, Mai W, Li M, Hu Y. Association between prediabetes and risk of cardiovascular disease and all cause mortality: systematic review and meta-analysis. *BMJ.* 2016;355:i5953.

Hubert HB, Feinleib M, McNamara PM, Castelli WP. Obesity as an independent risk factor for cardiovascular disease: a 26-year follow-up of participants in the Framingham Heart Study. *Circulation.* 1983;67:968-77.

Jousilahti P, Tuomilehto J, Vartiainen E, Pekkanen J, Puska P. Body weight, cardiovascular risk factors, and coronary mortality. 15-year follow-up of middle-aged men and women in eastern Finland. *Circulation. 1996;;93:1372-9.*

Kahn R, Buse J, Ferrannini E, Stern M: The metabolic syndrome: time for a critical appraisal: joint statement from the American Diabetes Association and the European Association for the Study of Diabetes. *Diabetes Care.* 28:2289-2304, 2005.

Kampoli AM, Tousoulis D, Briasoulis A, Latsios G, Papageorgiou N, Stefanadis C. Potential pathogenic inflammatory mechanisms of endothelial dysfunction induced by type 2 diabetes mellitus. *Curr Pharm Des.* 2011;17:4147–4158.

Kamstrup PR, Tybjaerg-Hansen A, Steffensen R, Nordestgaard BG. Genetically elevated lipoprotein(a) and increased risk of myocardial infarction. *J Am Med Assoc* 2009; 301: 2331–2339.

Kang HS, Gutin B, Barbeau P, Litaker MS, Allison J, Le NA. Low-density lipoprotein particle size, central obesity, cardiovascular fitness, and insulin resistance syndrome markers in obese youths. *Int J Obes Relat Metab Disord.* 2002;26:1030-5.

Kannel WB, Castelli WP, Gordon T, McNamara PM. Serum cholesterol, lipoproteins, and the risk of coronary heart disease. The Framingham study. *Ann Intern Med.* 1971;74:1-12.

Kannel WB, Castelli WP, McNamara PM, McKee PA, Feinleib M. Role of blood pressure in the development of congestive heart failure. The Framingham study. *N Engl J Med.* 1972;287:781-7.

Kannel WB. Role of blood pressure in cardiovascular disease: the Framingham Study. *Angiology.* 1975; 26(1 Pt. 1):1-14.

Khera AV, Demler OV, Adelman SJ, Collins HL, Glynn RJ, Ridker PM, Rader DJ, Mora S. Cholesterol Efflux Capacity, High-Density Lipoprotein Particle Number,and Incident Cardiovascular Events: An Analysis From the JUPITER Trial (Justification for the Use of Statins in Prevention: An Intervention Trial Evaluating Rosuvastatin). *Circulation.* 2017;135(25):2494-2504.

King GL, Park K, Li Q. Selective Insulin Resistance and the Development of Cardiovascular Diseases in Diabetes: The 2015 Edwin Bierman Award Lecture. *Diabetes.* 2016;65:1462-71.

Kizub IV, Klymenko KI, Soloviev AI. Protein kinase C in enhanced vascular tone in diabetes mellitus. *Int J Cardiol.* 2014;174:230-42.

Kougias P, Chai H, Lin PH, Yao Q, Lumsden AB, Chen C. Effects of adipocyte-derived cytokines on endothelial functions: implication of vascular disease. *J. Surg. Res.* 2005; 126, 121-129.

Kramer CK, Zinman B, Retnakaran R. Are metabolically healthy overweight and obesity benign conditions?: A systematic review and meta-analysis. *Ann Intern Med.* 2013;159:758-69.

Lakić D, Tasić L, Kos M. Economic burden of cardiovascular diseases in Serbia. *Vojnosanit Pregl.* 2014;71:137-43.

Lakka HM, Laaksonen DE, Lakka TA, Niskanen LK, Kumpusalo E, Tuomilehto J, Salonen JT: The metabolic syndrome and total and cardiovascular disease mortality in middle-aged men. *JAMA* 288:2709-2716, 2002.

Lanas F, Avezum A, Bautista LE, Diaz R, Luna M, Islam S, Yusuf S; INTERHEART Investigators in Latin America. Risk factors for acute myocardial infarction in Latin America: the INTERHEART Latin American study. *Circulation.* 2007;115:1067-74.

Lau DC, Dhillon B, Yan H, Szmitko PE, Verma S. Adipokines: molecular links between obesity and atheroslcerosis. 2005 *Am. J. Physiol. Heart Circ. Physiol.* 288(5), H2031-H2041.

Lee AK, Warren B, Lee CJ, McEvoy JW, Matsushita K, Huang ES, Sharrett AR, Coresh J, Selvin E. The association of severe hypoglycemia with incident cardiovascular events and mortality in adults with type 2 diabetes. *Diabetes Care* 2018; 41, 104–111.

Lee AS, Xi Y, Lai CH, Chen WY, Peng HY, Chan HC, Chen CH, Chang KC. Human electronegative low-density lipoprotein modulates cardiac repolarization via LOX-1-mediated alteration of sarcolemmal ion channels. *Sci Rep.* 2017;7:10889.

Lewis GF, Uffelman KD, Szeto LW, Steiner G. Effects of acute hyperinsulinemia on VLDL triglyceride and VLDL apoB production in normal weight and obese individuals. *Diabetes.* 1993;42:833-42.

Li C, Ford ES, Zhao G, Kahn HS, Mokdad AH. Waist-to-thigh ratio and diabetes among US adults: the Third National Health and Nutrition Examination Survey. *Diabetes Res Clin Pract.* 2010;89:79-87.

Li Q, Zhang Z, Du R. Association analysis between endothelial function related factors and coronary artery stenosis degree in coronary heart disease patients with type 2 diabetes mellitus. *J Pediatric Endocrinol Metab.* 2012;25:711–716.

Lim RB, Chen C, Naidoo N, Gay G, Tang WE, Seah D, Chen R, Tan NC, Lee J, Tai ES, Chia KS, Lim WY. Anthropometrics indices of obesity, and all-cause and cardiovascular disease-related mortality, in an Asian cohort with type 2 diabetes mellitus. *Diabetes Metab.* 2015;41:291-300.

Linder L, Kiowski W, Buhler FR, et al. Indirect evidence for release of endothelium-derived relaxing factor in human forearm circulation in vivo: blunted response in essential hypertension. *Circulation.* 1990; 81:1762–1767.

Long-Term Intervention with Pravastatin in Ischaemic Disease (LIPID) Study Group. Prevention of cardiovascular events and death with pravastatin in patients with coronary heart disease and a broad range of initial cholesterol levels. *N Engl J Med.* 1998;339:1349-57.

Lorenzo C, Williams K, Hunt KJ, Haffner SM. The National Cholesterol Education Program - Adult Treatment Panel III, International Diabetes Federation, and World Health Organization definitions of the metabolic syndrome as predictors of incident cardiovascular disease and diabetes. *Diabetes Care.* 2007;30:8-13.

Lu J, Jiang W, Yang JH, Chang PY, Walterscheid JP, Chen HH, Marcelli M, Tang D, Lee YT, Liao WS, Yang CY, Chen CH. Electronegative LDL impairs vascular endothelial cell integrity in diabetes by disrupting fibroblast growth factor 2 (FGF2) autoregulation. *Diabetes.* 2008; 57:158-66.

Makimattila S, Virkamaki A, Groop PH, Cockcroft J, Utriainen T, Fagerudd J, Yki-Jarvinen H. Chronic hyperglycemia impairs endothelial function and insulin sensitivity via different mechanisms in insulin-dependent diabetes mellitus. *Circulation.* 1996;94:1276–1282.

Mandavia CH, Aroor AR, Demarco VG, Sowers JR. Molecular and metabolic mechanisms of cardiac dysfunction in diabetes. *Life Sci.* 2013;92:601–608.

Marso SP, Bain SC, Consoli A, Eliaschewitz FG, Jódar E, Leiter LA, Lingvay I, Rosenstock J, Seufert J, Warren ML, Woo V, Hansen O, Holst AG, Pettersson J, Vilsbøll T; SUSTAIN-6 Investigators. Semaglutide and Cardiovascular outcomes in patients with type 2 Diabetes. *N Engl J Med.* 2016;375:1834-1844.

Marso SP, Daniels GH, Brown-Frandsen K, Kristensen P, Mann JF, Nauck MA, Nissen SE, Pocock S, Poulter NR, Ravn LS, Steinberg WM, Stockner M, Zinman B,Bergenstal RM, Buse JB; LEADER Steering Committee; LEADER Trial Investigators. Liraglutide and Cardiovascular Outcomes in Type 2 Diabetes. *N Engl J Med.* 2016; 375:311-22.

Marx N, Silbernagel G, Brandenburg V, Burgmaier M, Kleber ME, Grammer TB, Winkelmann BR, Boehm BO, März W. C-peptide levels are associated with mortality and cardiovascular mortality in patients undergoing angiography: the LURIC study. *Diabetes Care* 2013; 36:708-14.

Masters RK, Reither EN, Powers DA, Yang YC, Burger AE, Link BG. The impact of obesity on US mortality levels: the importance of age and cohort factors in population estimates. *Am J Public Health.* 2013;103:1895-901.

McAloon CJ, Boylan LM, Hamborg T, Stallard N, Osman F, Lim PB, Hayat SA. The changing face of cardiovascular disease 2000-2012: An analysis of the world health organisation global health estimates data. *Int J Cardiol.* 2016;224:256-264.

McCarron P, Smith GD, Okasha M, McEwen J. Blood pressure in young adulthood and mortality from cardiovascular disease. *Lancet.* 2000;355(9213):1430-1.

McQueen MJ, Hawken S, Wang X, Ounpuu S, Sniderman A, Probstfield J, Steyn K, Sanderson JE, Hasani M, Volkova E, Kazmi K, Yusuf S;

INTERHEART study investigators. Lipids, lipoproteins, and apolipoproteins as risk markers of myocardial infarction in 52 countries (the INTERHEART study): a case-control study. *Lancet.* 2008; 372(9634):224-33.

Mehta S, Ghosh S, Sander S, Kuti E, Mountford WK. Differences in All-Cause Health Care Utilization and Costs in a Type 2 Diabetes Mellitus Population with and Without a History of Cardiovascular Disease. *J Manag Care Spec Pharm.* 2018;24:280-290.

Min JY, Min KB. Serum C-peptide levels and risk of death among adults without diabetes mellitus. *CMAJ.* 2013;185:E402-8.

Montagnani M, Ravichandran LV, Chen H, Esposito DL, Quon MJ. Insulin receptor substrate-1 and phosphoinositide-dependent kinase-1 are required for insulin-stimulated production of nitric oxide in endothelial cells. *Mol Endocrinol.* 2002;16:1931-42.

Muniyappa R, Sowers JR. Role of insulin resistance in endothelial dysfunction. *Rev Endocr Metab Disord.* 2013;14:5-12.

Navab M, Imes SS, Hama SY, Hough GP, Ross LA, Bork RW, Valente AJ, Berliner JA, Drinkwater DC, Laks H, et al. Monocyte transmigration induced by modification of low density lipoprotein in cocultures of human aortic wall cells is due to induction of monocyte chemotactic protein 1 synthesis and is abolished by high density lipoprotein. *J Clin Invest.* 1991;88:2039-46.

Neal B, Perkovic V, Mahaffey KW, de Zeeuw D, Fulcher G, Erondu N, Shaw W, Law G, Desai M, Matthews DR; CANVAS Program Collaborative Group. Canagliflozin and Cardiovascular and Renal Events in Type 2 Diabetes. *N Engl J Med.* 2017;377:644-657.

Nestel PJ, Barnes EH, Tonkin AM, Simes J, Fournier M, White HD, Colquhoun DM, Blankenberg S, Sullivan DR. Plasma lipoprotein(a) concentration predicts future coronary and cardiovascular events in patients with stable coronary heart disease. *Arterioscler Thromb Vasc Biol.* 2013;33:2902-8.

Newens KJ, Thompson AK, Jackson KG, Williams CM. Endothelial function and insulin sensitivity during acute non-esterified fatty acid elevation: Effects of fat composition and gender. *Nutr Metab Cardiovasc Dis.* 2015;25:575-81.

Nicholls SJ, Tuzcu EM, Kalidindi S, Wolski K, Moon KW, Sipahi I, Schoenhagen P, Nissen SE. Effect of diabetes on progression of coronary atherosclerosis and arterial remodeling: a pooled analysis of 5 intravascular ultrasound trials. *J Am Coll Cardiol.* 2008;52:255-62.

Nordestgaard BG, Benn M, Schnohr P, Tybjaerg-Hansen A. Nonfasting triglycerides and risk of myocardial infarction, ischemic heart disease, and death in men and women. *JAMA.* 2007;298:299-308.

Orencia AJ, Daviglus ML, Dyer AR, Walsh M, Greenland P, Stamler J. One-hour postload plasma glucose and risks of fatal coronary heart disease and stroke among nondiabetic men and women: the Chicago Heart Association Detection Project in Industry (CHA) Study. *J Clin Epidemiol.* 1997;50:1369-76.

Organization WH and UNAIDS. *Prevention of cardiovascular disease*: World Health Organization; 2007.

Pajunen P, Rissanen H, Härkänen T, Jula A, Reunanen A, Salomaa V. The metabolic syndrome as a predictor of incident diabetes and cardiovascular events in the Health 2000 Study. *Diabetes Metab.* 2010; 36:395-401.

Panza JA, Casino PR, Kilcoyne CM, Quyyumi AA. Role of endothelium-derived nitric oxide in the abnormal endothelium-dependent vascular relaxation of patients with essential hypertension. *Circulation.* 1993; 87:1468–1474.

Panza JA, Quyyumi AA, Brush JE Jr, Epstein SE. Abnormal endothelium-dependent vascular relaxation in patients with essential hypertension. *N Engl J Med.* 1990;323:22–27.

Park HK, Kwak MK, Kim HJ, Ahima RS. Linking resistin, inflammation, and cardiometabolic diseases. *Korean J Intern Med.* 2017;32:239-247.

Perassolo MS, Almeida JC, Steemburgo T, Dall'Alba V, de Mello VD, Zelmanovitz T, de Azevedo MJ, Gross JL. Endothelial dysfunction and serum fatty acid composition in patients with type 2 diabetes mellitus. *Metabolism.* 2008;57:1167-72.

Pieters M, van Zyl DG, Rheeder P, Jerling JC, Loots du T, van der Westhuizen FH, Gottsche LT, Weisel JW. Glycation of fibrinogen in uncontrolled diabetic patients and the effects of glycaemic control on fibrinogen glycation. *Thromb Res* 2007;120:439-446.

Pilz S, Scharnagl H, Tiran B, Seelhorst U, Wellnitz B, Boehm BO, Schaefer JR, März W. Free fatty acids are independently associated with all-cause and cardiovascular mortality in subjects with coronary artery disease. *J Clin Endocrinol Metab.* 2006;91:2542-7.

Pirro M, Mauriège P, Tchernof A, Cantin B, Dagenais GR, Després JP, Lamarche B. Plasma free fatty acid levels and the risk of ischemic heart disease in men: prospective results from the Québec Cardiovascular Study. *Atherosclerosis.* 2002;160:377-84.

Pischon T, Girman CJ, Sacks FM, Rifai N, Stampfer MJ, Rimm EB. Non-high-density lipoprotein cholesterol and apolipoprotein B in the prediction of coronary heart disease in men. *Circulation.* 2005; 112:3375-83.

Pontiroli AE, Pizzocri P, Koprivec D, Vedani P, Marchi M, Arcelloni C, Paroni R, Esposito K, Giugliano D: Body weight and glucose metabolism have a different effect on circulating levels of ICAM-1, E-selectin, and endothelin-1 in humans. *Eur J Endocrinol* 2004;150: 195–200.

Pyörälä K, Ballantyne CM, Gumbiner B, Lee MW, Shah A, Davies MJ, Mitchel YB, Pedersen TR, Kjekshus J; Scandinavian Simvastatin Survival Study (4S). Reduction of cardiovascular events by simvastatin in nondiabetic coronary heart disease patients with and without the metabolic syndrome: subgroup analyses of the Scandinavian Simvastatin Survival Study (4S). *Diabetes Care.* 2004;27:1735-40.

Pyorala M, Miettinen, H., Laasko, M., and Pyorala, K. Hyperinsulinemia predicts coronary heart disease risk in healthy middle-aged men: the 22-year follow-up results of the Helsinki Policemen Study. *Circulation* 1998; 98, 398-404.

Rawshani A, Rawshani A, Franzén S, Eliasson B, Svensson AM, Miftaraj M, McGuire DK, Sattar N, Rosengren A, Gudbjörnsdottir S. Mortality and Cardiovascular Disease in Type 1 and Type 2 Diabetes. *N Engl J Med.* 2017;13;376:1407-1418.

Ray KK, Cannon CP, Braunwald E: Recent trials of lipid lowering. *International Journal of Clinical Practice* 2007; 61, 1145-1159.

Rexrode KM, Carey VJ, Hennekens CH, Walters EE, Colditz GA, Stampfer MJ, Willett WC, Manson JE. Abdominal adiposity and coronary heart disease in women. *JAMA.* 1998;280:1843-8.

Saad MI, Abdelkhalek TM, Saleh MM, Kamel MA, Youssef M, Tawfik SH, Dominguez H. Insights into the molecular mechanisms of diabetes-induced endothelial dysfunction: focus on oxidative stress and endothelial progenitor cells. *Endocrine.* 2015;50:537-67.

Sapkota B, Shrestha SK, Poudel S. Association of activated partial thromboplastin time and fibrinogen level in patients with type II diabetes mellitus. *BMC Res Notes.* 2013;6:485.

Sarwar N, Danesh J, Eiriksdottir G, Sigurdsson G, Wareham N, Bingham S, Boekholdt SM, Khaw KT, Gudnason V. Triglycerides and the risk of coronary heart disease: 10,158 incident cases among 262,525 participants in 29 Western prospective studies. *Circulation.* 2007; 115:450-8.

Seligman BG, Biolo A, Polanczyk CA, Gross JL, Clausell N. Increased plasma levels of endothelin 1 and von Willebrand factor in patients with type 2 diabetes and dyslipidemia. *Diabetes Care.* 2000;23:1395–1400.

Sever PS, Dahlöf B, Poulter NR, Wedel H, Beevers G, Caulfield M, Collins R, Kjeldsen SE, Kristinsson A, McInnes GT, Mehlsen J, Nieminen M, O'Brien E, Ostergren J; ASCOT investigators. Prevention of coronary and stroke events with atorvastatin in hypertensive patients who have average or lower-than-average cholesterol concentrations, in the Anglo-Scandinavian Cardiac Outcomes Trial--Lipid Lowering Arm (ASCOT-LLA): a multicentre randomised controlled trial. *Lancet.* 2003; 361(9364):1149-58.

Shahim B, De Bacquer D, De Backer G, Gyberg V, Kotseva K, Mellbin L, Schnell O, Tuomilehto J, Wood D, Rydén L. The Prognostic Value of Fasting Plasma Glucose, Two-Hour Postload Glucose, and HbA(1c) in Patients With Coronary Artery Disease: A Report From EUROASPIRE

IV: A Survey From the European Society of Cardiology. *Diabetes Care.* 2017;40:1233-1240.

Sharrett AR, Ballantyne CM, Coady SA, Heiss G, Sorlie PD, Catellier D, Patsch W; Atherosclerosis Risk in Communities Study Group. Coronary heart disease prediction from lipoprotein cholesterol levels, triglycerides, lipoprotein(a), apolipoproteins A-I and B, and HDL density subfractions: The Atherosclerosis Risk in Communities (ARIC) Study. *Circulation.* 2001;104:1108–1113.

Sniderman AD, Thanassoulis G, Glavinovic T, Navar AM, Pencina M, Catapano A, Ference BA. Apolipoprotein B Particles and Cardiovascular Disease: A Narrative Review. *JAMA Cardiol.* 2019. [Epub ahead of print]

Song X, Yang B, Qiu F, Jia M, Fu G. High glucose and free fatty acids induce endothelial progenitor cell senescence via PGC-1α/SIRT1 signaling pathway. *Cell Biol Int.* 2017;41:1146-1159.

Song Z, Wang W, Li N, Yan S, Rong K, Lan T, Xia P. Sphingosine kinase 2 promotes lipotoxicity in pancreatic β-cells and the progression of diabetes. *FASEB J.* 2019;33:3636-3646.

Soria-Florido MT, Castañer O, Lassale C, Estruch R, Salas-Salvadó J, Martínez-González MÁ, Corella D, Ros E, Arós F, Elosua R, Lapetra J, Fiol M, Alonso-Gómez A, Gómez-Gracia E, Serra-Majem L, Pintó X, Bulló M, Ruiz-Canela M, Sorlí JV, Hernáez Á, Fitó M. Dysfunctional HDLs are Associated with a Greater Incidence of Acute Coronary Syndrome in a Population at High Cardiovascular Risk: A Nested-Case Control Study. *Circulation.* 2020. doi:10.1161/CIRCULATIONAHA. 119.041658.

SPRINT Research Group, Wright JT Jr, Williamson JD, Whelton PK, Snyder JK, Sink KM, Rocco MV, Reboussin DM, Rahman M, Oparil S, Lewis CE, Kimmel PL, Johnson KC, Goff DC Jr, Fine LJ, Cutler JA, Cushman WC, Cheung AK, Ambrosius WT. A Randomized Trial of Intensive versus Standard Blood-Pressure Control. *N Engl J Med.* 2015;373:2103-16.

Srivastava RAK. Dysfunctional HDL in diabetes mellitus and its role in the pathogenesis of cardiovascular disease. *Mol Cell Biochem.* 2018; 440:167-187.

Stamler J, Daviglus ML, Garside DB, Dyer AR, Greenland P, Neaton JD. Relationship of baseline serum cholesterol levels in 3 large cohorts of younger men to long-term coronary, cardiovascular, and all-cause mortality and to longevity. *JAMA* 2000;284:311-8.

Stamler J, Neaton JD, Wentworth DN. Blood pressure (systolic and diastolic) and risk of fatal coronary heart disease. *Hypertension.* 1989; 13(5Suppl):I2-12.

Stamler J, Vaccaro O, Neaton JD, Wentworth D. Diabetes, other risk factors, and 12-yr cardiovascular mortality for men screened in the Multiple Risk Factor Intervention Trial. *Diabetes Care.* 1993;16:434-44.

Stefan N, Häring HU, Hu FB, Schulze MB. Metabolically healthy obesity: epidemiology, mechanisms, and clinical implications. *Lancet Diabetes Endocrinol* 2013;1:152-62.

Steinberg HO, Paradisi G, Hook G, Crowder K, Cronin J, Baron AD. Free fatty acid elevation impairs insulin-mediated vasodilation and nitric oxide production. *Diabetes.* 2000; 49:1231-1238.

Steinberg HO, Tarshoby M, Monestel R, Hook G, Cronin J, Johnson A, Bayazeed B, Baron AD. Elevated circulating free fatty acid levels impair endothelium-dependent vasodilation. *J Clin Invest.* 1997; 100:1230-1239.

Tabara Y, Takahashi Y, Setoh K, Kawaguchi T, Gotoh N, Terao C, Yamada R, Kosugi S, Sekine A, Nakayama T, Matsuda F; Nagahama Study group. Synergistic association of elevated serum free fatty acid and glucose levels with large arterial stiffness in a general population: The Nagahama Study. *Metabolism.* 2016;65:66-72.

Tabit CE, Shenouda SM, Holbrook M, Fetterman JL, Kiani S, Frame AA, Kluge MA, Held A, Dohadwala MM, Gokce N, Farb MG, Rosenzweig J, Ruderman N, Vita JA, Hamburg NM. Protein kinase C-β contributes to impaired endothelial insulin signaling in humans with diabetes mellitus. *Circulation* 2013;127:86-95.

Taskinen MR, Nikkilä EA, Kuusi T, Harmo K. Lipoprotein lipase activity and serum lipoproteins in untreated type 2 (insulin-independent) diabetes associated with obesity. *Diabetologia.* 1982;22:46-50.

Thanassoulis G, Tardif JC, Huynh T. Meta-analysis of Randomized Controlled Trials Assessing the Impact of Proprotein Convertase Subtilisin/Kexin Type 9 Antibodies on Mortality and Cardiovascular Outcomes. *Am J Cardiol.* 201915;124(:1869-1875.

The National Institute of Health and Clinical Excellence. Hypertension in adults: diagnosis and management. *Guideline NG136.* 2019: https://www.nice.org.uk/guidance/ng136 (accessed 30th January 2020).

The Scandinavian Simvastatin Survival Study Group. Randomised trial of cholesterol lowering in 4444 patients with coronary heart disease: the Scandinavian Simvastatin Survival Study (4S). *Lancet.* 1994, 19; 344(8934):1383-9.

Third Report of the National Cholesterol Education Program (NCEP) Expert Panel on Detection, Evaluation, and Treatment of High Blood Cholesterol in Adults (Adult Treatment Panel III) *final report Circulation* 2002;106, 3143-3421.

Tomkin GH, Owens D. Insulin and lipoprotein metabolism with special reference to the diabetic state. *Diabetes Metab Rev.* 10:225 –252,1994.

Trpkovic A, Resanovic I, Stanimirovic J, Radak D, Mousa SA, Cenic-Milosevic D, Jevremovic D, Isenovic ER. Oxidized low-density lipoprotein as a biomarker of cardiovascular diseases. *Crit Rev Clin Lab Sci.* 2015;52:70-85.

Turner RC, Millns H, Neil HA, et al. Risk factors for coronary artery disease in non-insulin dependent diabetes mellitus: United Kingdom prospective diabetes study (UKPDS: 23) *BMJ.* 1998;316:823–828.

Turner RC, Millns H, Neil HA, Stratton IM, Manley SE, Matthews DR, Holman RR. Risk factors for coronary artery disease in non-insulin dependent diabetes mellitus: United Kingdom Prospective Diabetes Study (UKPDS: 23). *BMJ.* 1998;316(7134):823-8.

UK Prospective Diabetes Study (UKPDS) Group. Intensive blood-glucose control with sulphonylureas or insulin compared with conventional treatment and risk of complications in patients with type 2 diabetes (UKPDS 33). *Lancet.* 1998;352(9131):837-53.

Vaisar T, Couzens E, Hwang A, Russell M, Barlow CE, DeFina LF, Hoofnagle AN,Kim F. Type 2 diabetes is associated with loss of HDL endothelium protective functions. *PLoS One.* 2018;13:e0192616.

van Kruijsdijk RC, van der Graaf Y, Koffijberg H, de Borst GJ, Nathoe HM, Jaap Kappelle L, Visseren FL; SMART study group. Cause-specific mortality and years of life lost in patients with different manifestations of vascular disease. *Eur J Prev Cardiol.* 2016;23:160-9.

Van Lenten BJ, Hama SY, de Beer FC, Stafforini DM, McIntyre TM, Prescott SM, La Du BN, Fogelman AM, Navab M. Anti-inflammatory HDL Becomes pro-inflammatory during the acute phase response. Loss of protective effect of HDL against LDL oxidation in aortic wall cell cocultures. *J Clin Invest.* 1995;96:2758–2767.

Véricel E, Januel C, Carreras M, Moulin P, Lagarde M. Diabetic patients without vascular complications display enhanced basal platelet activation and decreased antioxidant status. *Diabetes.* 2004;53:1046-51.

Vokonas PS, Kannel WB, Cupples LA. Epidemiology and risk of hypertension in the elderly: the Framingham Study. *J Hypertens Suppl.* 1988;6:S3-9.

Wägner AM, Jorba O, Rigla M, Alonso E, Ordóñez-Llanos J. Pérez A. LDL-cholesterol/apolipoprotein B ratio is a good predictor of LDL phenotype B in type 2 diabetes. *Acta Diabetol.* 2002;39:215-20.

Wägner AM, Pérez A, Zapico E, Ordóñez-Llanos J. Non-HDL cholesterol and apolipoprotein B in the dyslipidemic classification of type 2 diabetic patients. *Diabetes Care.* 2003;26:2048-51.

Walldius G, Jungner I, Holme I, Aastveit AH, Kolar W, Steiner E. High apolipoprotein B, low apolipoprotein A-I, and improvement in the prediction of fatal myocardial infarction (AMORIS study): a prospective study. *Lancet.* 2001. 15:358(9298), 2026-3.

Wang A, Yang Y, Su Z, Yue W, Hao H, Ren L, Wang Y, Cao Y, Wang Y. Association of Oxidized Low-Density Lipoprotein With Prognosis of Stroke and Stroke Subtypes. *Stroke.* 2017;48:91-97.

Wang YC, Lee AS, Lu LS, Ke LY, Chen WY, Dong JW, Lu J, Chen Z, Chu CS, Chan HC, Kuzan TY, Tsai MH, Hsu WL, Dixon RAF, Sawamura T, Chang KC, Chen CH. Human electronegative LDL induces mitochondrial dysfunction and premature senescence of vascular cells in vivo. *Aging Cell.* 2018;e12792.

Wannamethee SG, Shaper AG, Lennon L et al. Metabolic syndrome vs Framingham Risk Score for prediction of coronary heart disease, stroke, and type 2 diabetes mellitus. *Arch Intern Med.* 2005; 165: 2644–2650.

Weber MA, Bakris GL, Dahlöf B, Pitt B, Velazquez E, Gupte J, Lefkowitz M, Hester A, Shi V, Weir M, Kjeldsen S, Massie B, Nesbitt S, Ofili E, Jamerson K. Baseline characteristics in the Avoiding Cardiovascular events through Combination therapy in Patients Living with Systolic Hypertension (ACCOMPLISH) trial: a hypertensive population at high cardiovascular risk. *Blood Press.* 2007;16:13-9.

Wildman RP, Muntner P, Reynolds K, McGinn AP, Rajpathak S, Wylie-Rosett J, Sowers MR. The obese without cardiometabolic risk factor clustering and the normal weight with cardiometabolic risk factor clustering: prevalence and correlates of 2 phenotypes among the US population (NHANES 1999-2004). *Arch Intern Med.* 2008;168:1617-24.

Wilson PW, Abbott RD, Castelli WP. High density lipoprotein cholesterol and mortality. The Framingham Heart Study. *Arteriosclerosis.* 1988; 8(6):737-41.

Wilson PW, D'Agostino RB, Levy D, Belanger AM, Silbershatz H, Kannel WB. Prediction of coronary heart disease using risk factor categories. *Circulation.* 1998;97:1837–1847.

Witteles RM, Fowler MB. Insulin-resistant cardiomyopathy clinical evidence, mechanisms, and treatment options. *J Am Coll Cardiol.* 2008;51:93–102.

Wiviott SD, Raz I, Bonaca MP, Mosenzon O, Kato ET, Cahn A, Silverman MG, Zelniker TA, Kuder JF, Murphy SA, Bhatt DL, Leiter LA, McGuire DK, Wilding JPH, Ruff CT, Gause-Nilsson IAM, Fredriksson M, Johansson PA, Langkilde AM, Sabatine MS; DECLARE–TIMI 58

Investigators. Dapagliflozin and cardiovascular Outcomes in type 2 Diabetes. *N Engl J Med.* 2019;380:347-357.

World Health Organization (2000). 'Controlling the global obesity epidemic', World Health Organization. file:///C:/Users/user/Downloads/WHO_TRS_894.pdf (accessed 20th January 2020).

World Health Organization: *Definition, Diagnosis and Classification of Diabetes Mellitus and Its Complications: Report of a WHO Consultation.* Geneva, World Health Org., 1999.

Xu H, Barnes GT, Yang Q et al. Chronic inflammation in fat plays a crucial role in the development of obesity-related insulin resistance. *J. Clin. Invest.* 2003; 112, 1821-1830.

Yamagishi S, Nakamura N, Suematsu M, Kaseda K, Matsui T. Advanced Glycation End Products: A Molecular Target for Vascular Complications in Diabetes. *Mol Med.* 2015;21 Suppl 1:S32-40.

Yano Y, Reis JP, Lewis CE, Sidney S, Pletcher MJ, Bibbins-Domingo K, Navar AM, Peterson ED, Bancks MP, Kanegae H, Gidding SS, Muntner P, Lloyd-Jones DM. Association of Blood Pressure Patterns in Young Adulthood With Cardiovascular Disease and Mortality in Middle Age. *JAMA Cardiol.* 2020 Jan 22.

Yano Y, Stamler J, Garside DB, Daviglus ML, Franklin SS, Carnethon MR, Liu K, Greenland P, Lloyd-Jones DM. Isolated systolic hypertension in young and middle-aged adults and 31-year risk for cardiovascular mortality: the Chicago Heart Association Detection Project in Industry study. *J Am Coll Cardiol.* 2015;65:327-35.

Ying W, Fu W, Lee YS, Olefsky JM. The role of macrophages in obesity-associated islet inflammation and β-cell abnormalities. *Nat Rev Endocrinol.* 2020;16:81-90.

Yusuf S, Hawken S, Ounpuu S, Bautista L, Franzosi MG, Commerford P, Lang CC, Rumboldt Z, Onen CL, Lisheng L, Tanomsup S, Wangai P Jr, Razak F, Sharma AM, Anand SS; INTERHEART Study Investigators. Obesity and the risk of myocardial infarction in 27,000 participants from 52 countries: a case-control study. *Lancet.* 2005;366(9497):1640-9.

Yusuf S, Hawken S, Ounpuu S, Dans T, Avezum A, Lanas F, McQueen M, Budaj A, Pais P, Varigos J, Lisheng L; INTERHEART Study

Investigators. Effect of potentially modifiable risk factors associated with myocardial infarction in 52 countries (the INTERHEART study): case-control study. *Lancet.* 2004. 11-17;364(9438):937-52.

Yusuf S, Hawken S, Ounpuu S, Dans T, Avezum A, Lanas F, McQueen M, Budaj A, Pais P, Varigos J, Lisheng L, for the INTERHEART Study Investigators. Effect of potentially modifiable risk factors associated with AMI in 52 countries (the INTERHEART study): case-control study. *Lancet.* 2004; 364:937–952.

Zhang Q, Ai Y, Dong H, Wang J, Xu L. Circulating Oxidized Low-Density Lipoprotein is a Strong Risk Factor for the Early Stage of Coronary Heart Disease. *IUBMB Life.* 2019;71:277-282.

Zinman B, Wanner C, Lachin JM, Fitchett D, Bluhmki E, Hantel S, Mattheus M, Devins T, Johansen OE, Woerle HJ, Broedl UC, Inzucchi SE; EMPA-REG OUTCOME Investigators. Empagliflozin, Cardiovascular outcomes, and mortality in type 2 diabetes. *N Engl J Med.* 2015;373:2117-28.

Zoungas S, Patel A, Chalmers J, de Galan BE, Li Q, Billot L, Woodward M, Ninomiya T, Neal B, MacMahon S, Grobbee DE, Kengne AP, Marre M, Heller S; ADVANCE Collaborative Group. Severe hypoglycemia and risks of vascular events and death. *N Engl J Med.* 2010;363:1410-8.

In: Cardiometabolic Diseases and Risk Factors ISBN: 978-1-53618-111-1
Editor: Patrick Ralston © 2020 Nova Science Publishers, Inc.

Chapter 2

CARDIO-METABOLIC RISK FACTORS IN POLYCYSTIC OVARY SYNDROME

Fahimeh Ramezani Tehrani[1,*], *MD*
and Samira Behboudi-Gandevani[2], *PhD*

[1]Reproductive Endocrinology Research Center, Research Institute for Endocrine Sciences, Shahid Beheshti University of Medical Sciences, Tehran, Iran
[2]Faculty of Nursing and Health Sciences, Nord University, Bodø, Norway

ABSTRACT

Polycystic ovary syndrome (PCOS) is one of the most common endocrine disorders with an estimated prevalence of 7% to 14% among reproductive-aged women. Although the exact underlying etiology of PCOS is not entirely clear, however, evidence has shown that insulin resistance, hyperandrogenemia and adipose tissue dysregulation play key roles on its pathogenesis. The syndrome is recognized as a cardio-metabolic disorder. Data have shown that traditional cardiovascular and

---

[*] Corresponding Author's Email: fah.tehrani@gmail.com; ramezani@endocrine.ac.ir.

metabolic risk factors including hypertension, dyslipidemia, metabolic syndrome, obesity and central obesity, glucose intolerance and diabetes are more prevalent among PCOS patients. In addition, subclinical cardiovascular markers such as coronary artery calcium scores, C-reactive protein, carotid intima-media thickness and endothelial dysfunction are more likely to be increased in women with PCOS. Nevertheless, there is much more controversy regarding whether cardio-metabolic events are increased in PCOS in later life, leaving many issues regarding cardiovascular and metabolic events unresolved. This chapter will discuss the literature on PCOS and cardio-metabolic risk factors and provides recommendations that would be helpful for healthcare provider and policy makers in the monitoring and management of these risk factors in PCOS population. Treatment options are beyond the scope of this chapter.

Keywords: cardio-metabolic risk factors, polycystic ovary syndrome (PCOS), cardio vascular diseases (CVD)

1. INTRODUCTION

Polycystic ovary syndrome (PCOS) is the most common endocrine disorder, with an estimated prevalence of 7% to 20% among women of reproductive age [1-3]. Heterogeneous by nature, the syndrome is characterized by a combination of signs and symptoms of ovarian dysfunction (including oligo/anovulation, and/or polycystic ovarian morphology (PCOM)) and androgen excess (including hyperandrogenemia and/or hyperandrogenism), after the exclusion of other related disorders [4, 5].

The exact underlying etiology and pathogenesis of PCOS remains largely unknown, but it seems to be a complex interactions between multifactorial components of genetic, epigenetic, environmental and lifestyle factors [6, 7]. The imbalance in sex hormones and insulin resistance (IR) are considered to be a main factor of the reproductive and metabolic abnormalities in PCOS [8, 9]. Insulin resistance with compensatory increased insulin production contributes to hyperandro-genemia due to the augmentation of ovarian androgen production and the inhibition of hepatic sex hormone-binding globulin secretion [5]. Moreover, PCOS is closely linked to adipose tissue dysregulation [10], which is characterized by hypertrophic adipocytes and impairments in lipolysis and insulin action [11, 12]. Further, chronic low grade inflammation [13, 14] and excessive formation of oxidative stress [15, 16] have been actively implicated in the etiology of the syndrome.

Data have shown that traditional cardiovascular/metabolic risk factors such as obesity and central obesity [17, 18], increased carotid intima media thickness [19, 20] and coronary artery calcifications [21] are more common among women with PCOS compared with the age-matched women without the syndrome.

However, despite the presence of cardiovascular risk factors and increased surrogate markers of cardiovascular disease, it is not clearly understood whether PCOS patients have accelerated atherosclerosis or other cardiovascular events and also greater mortality, the latter mainly because of a lack of long term endpoint studies.

This chapter addresses, summarizes, and discusses salient data from the existing literature, including gaps and uncertainties, aspects, and mechanisms related to the spectrum of adverse cardiometabolic profile factors in women with PCOS.

This chapter outlines, summarizes, and discusses salient data from the existing literature, including gaps and uncertainties, latest advances and current limitations and mechanisms related to the spectrum of cardiometabolic aspects in PCOS.

1.1. Definition of PCOS

Some sets of criteria for diagnosis have been proposed for PCOS. At the first time, National Institutes of Health (NIH) in 1990 introduce the PCOS diagnosis criteria including only presence of clinical and/or biochemical hyperandrogenism and oligo/anovulation [22]. Later, two international consensus have developed adult diagnostic criteria that broaden the definition beyond NIH criteria by incorporating the presence of polycystic ovary morphology [23, 24] as a diagnostic criterion for PCOS. Rotterdam criteria in 2003 are the broadest and encompass all combinations and require two of three features including oligo/anovulation, clinical and/or biochemical hyperandrogenism and PCOM in ultrasound assessment [25]. Androgen Excess-PCOS (AE-PCOS) Society criteria in 2006 encompass otherwise unexplained hyperandrogenism with either oligo/anovulation or PCOM [23].

In addition, the presentation of PCOS reflects at least four possible phenotypes (Phenotypes A–D) depending on the presence or absence of three general features of oligo-anovulation, androgen excess and polycystic ovarian morphology) [26]

- Phenotype A: Hirsutism/hyperandrogenemia + Ovulatory dysfunction + Polycystic ovaries (classic combination of all the reproductive endocrine features)
- Phenotype B: Hirsutism/hyperandrogenemia + Ovulatory dysfunction
- Phenotype C: Hirsutism/hyperandrogenemia + Polycystic ovaries
- Phenotype D: Ovulatory dysfunction + Polycystic ovaries

Whether these phenotypes represent a continuum of the same condition, but PCOS phenotypes with hyperandrogenism and oligo/ anovulation had the worst metabolic presentations in terms of insulin resistance, diabetes, obesity, metabolic syndrome and cardiovascular disease [27-29]. However, further characterization of PCOS phenotypic differences is an important area for ongoing research.

The diagnosis of PCOS in adolescent female populations is complicating, since adolescence is a transitional stage of physical and psychological development and functional variations in the hypothalamic-pituitary-ovarian axis during normal puberty leads to changes in reproductive hormones and menstrual patterns that mimic some of the features of PCOS. Moreover, many of the PCOS features may evolve over time and change during the first few years after menarche. There is no consensus on precise diagnosis of PCOS in adolescents [30] Therefore, international consensus have endorsed more stringent criteria including using all three components of the Rotterdam criteria [31] or using NIH criteria for diagnosis of PCOS in adolescents [32]. However, precise definition of PCOS in adolescent is essential, since associated cardiometabolic morbidity such as obesity, insulin resistance and dyslipidemia may benefit from early intervention approaches.

1.2. Pathogenesis of Polycystic Ovary Syndrome

PCOS is a multifactorial disease. The interaction between genetic predisposition, intra-uterine (prenatal) and postnatal environmental factors may comprise in development of PCOS [6, 7, 33].

Although, the genes that are involved in the etiology of the syndrome have not been fully understood yet, the role of genetic factors in PCOS is strongly supported [34-38]. Studies of twins in which women with monozygotic twin sisters affected by PCOS and also first-degree relatives of women with PCOS were shown to have higher the risk of developing PCOS features and metabolic disturbances, which suggests a genetic background effect and familial condition. Although there are low external validity, gene variants of lots of coding genes associated with the clinical and laboratory features of PCOS have been demonstrated in these populations [39]. In addition, some genes have shown altered expression indicating that the genetic abnormality in PCOS affects signal transduction pathways regulating insulin, gonadotrophin and steroid hormones action and production as well as energy homeostasis, chronic inflammation and others [40].

In addition, environmental factors potentially could involve in PCOS development which are classified as prenatal intra-uterine developmental programming and postnatal factors [41-43]. Evidence suggests that environmental stimuli can both mimic hormonal actions and activate pre-existing, predisposing factors that trigger the endocrine activity characteristic of PCOS [6]. Glucocorticoids excess during critical period of fetal development, either by the fetal origin (resulting from fetal hypoxia and IUGR) [44, 45] or maternal source (resulting from elevation of endogenous or exogenous maternal androgen levels during pregnancy) [46, 47] may related to PCOS developmental programming. It may lead to functional changes in organs, endocrine pathways and subsequently clinical, metabolic and reproductive changes during postnatal life [48]. In this respect, it is demonstrated that sexual function of women whose mothers also had PCOS and therefore potentially may had prenatal androgen exposure, was significantly decreased compared to women whose mothers did not [49]. In addition, postnatal factors including diet and nutrition, obesity, sedentary lifestyle, environmental toxins, medications and social and economic factors may play a role in development of PCOS [42].

1.3. PCOS and Traditional Cardio-Metabolic Risk Factors

1.3.1. Insulin Resistance, Glucose Intolerance and Diabetes Mellitus

Insulin resistance play a key role in the metabolic manifestations among women with PCOS which is independent of BMI and obesity [50]. The prevalence of IR among women with PCOS is estimated around 30% and 70%, based on the women's age, obesity status and ethnicity [51]. In this respect, older age, higher BMI and Hispanic ethnicity exacerbates IR to a greater extent in women with than those without PCOS, irrespective of the definition used [8, 50, 52]. However, it is well documented that high testosterone and low sex hormone-binding globulin (SHBG) concentrations are independently associated with IR [53-55]. It has been shown that the PCOS phenotypes with hyperandrogenism are strongly associated with insulin resistant, irrespective of BMI or central adiposity [9, 56, 57]. Additionally, it seems that despite common genetic variations at the diabetes related loci in PCOS and non PCOS women, the association between IR and diabetogenic polymorphisms may be affected by PCOS status [58]

There are several underlying mechanisms have been proposed for the development of IR in PCOS including (i) an increase in serine phosphorylation that causes post-binding defects in insulin signalling [59], and disturbances in the tyrosine phosphorylation of insulin receptors and insulin receptor substrate-1 that affects metabolic pathways in classic insulin targets mainly adipocytes, skeletal muscles and ovaries [59], (ii) reduced insulin receptor-β abundance in omental adipose tissue, reduced glucose transporter 4 (GLUT4) in subcutaneous adipocytes, both leading to reduction in glucose uptake, (iii) reduced hepatic clearance of insulin, (iv) mitochondrial dysfunction, constitutive activation of serine kinases in the mitogen-activated protein kinase/extracellular signal-regulated kinases pathway [59], (v) genetic disruption of insulin signalling in the central nervous system (vi) chronic low-grade inflammation with increased tumor necrosis factor-alpha (TNF-α) secretion from mononuclear cells [60, 61] (vii) increased iron tissue depots due to chronic oligo/anovulation that lead to impair insulin secretion by oxidative damage of β cells and decrease insulin clearance and muscle glucose uptake [62, 63]. However, increased level of insulin due to the both increased insulin production and reduced insulin clearance in liver, could induce higher androgen secretion. Hyperandrogenemia *per se* could change insulin action in the target tissues leading to increase visceral adiposity in PCOS women [64].

It should be noted that IR and hyperinsulinemia may play further important roles in the modulation of cardiovascular risk. Insulin resistance may lead to disturbance in natriuretic peptides (NP) which are secreted from cardiomyocytes and directly influence blood pressure, body fluid homeostasis, and various metabolic functions including lipolytic activity [65, 66]. Insulin increases the expression of NP clearance receptor in adipose tissue, independent of glycemia [67-69].

Although there is some variability in reports of the prevalence of prediabetes and DM among women with PCOS, most studies agree that women with PCOS have a higher prevalence of impaired fasting glucose (IFG), impaired glucose tolerance (IGT), and DM, especially among the obese. [3, 70-73]. In a prospective study of 254 PCOS women, it is showed that that 31% of PCOS patients had impaired glucose intolerance, and 7.5% had diabetes; a 3- to 7-fold higher than the age-comparable population, and around a 2-fold higher risk compared with age- and BMI-comparable women with normal cycles [74]. In another long term population based prospective study among 178 women with PCOS and 1524 eumenorrheic, non-hirsute, healthy women, it is showed that the risk of developing diabetes and prediabetes in young women with PCOS is 4.9 and 1.7 times higher, respectively, than in the general female population after adjustment for potential related confounders. In contrast, those hazard differences between PCOS and controls disappeared in their late reproductive years [70]. A recent systematic review and meta-analysis of 40 quality studies found women with PCOS had an increased prevalence of impaired glucose tolerance (IGT) (OR = 3.26, 95% CI: 2.17-4.90) and T2DM (OR = 2.87, 95% CI: 1.44-5.72), which differed by ethnicity (for IGT, Asia: 5-fold, the Americas: 4-fold and Europe: 3-fold), was higher with obesity [73].

Taken together, the findings support close monitoring, with screening for T2DM in women with PCOS [75]. In this respect, the Endocrine Society [32] and ESHRE/ASRM [25] recommended the use of OGTT in all adolescents and adult women with PCOS. Nevertheless, there is no evidence on the optimal time for serial screening, but it has been arbitrarily suggested every three to five years, except for an earlier worsening in clinical symptomatology [32]. Reciprocally, the European Society of Endocrinology (ESE) in 2014 endorsed an oral glucose tolerance test (OGTT) in all obese and lean women with PCOS older than 40 years, with a positive history of GDM or family history of T2DM [76].

1.3.2. Dyslipidemia

There are many studies showed that dyslipidemia is one of the common feature of metabolic disturbances among women with PCOS [59, 77]. A meta-analysis in 2011 reported that PCOS patients had 26.39 (95% CI 17.24, 35.54) mg/dl higher TG levels, 6.41 (95% CI 3.69, 9.14) mg/dl lower HDL-C and 18.82 (95% CI 15.53, 22.11) mg/dl higher non- HDL-C levels compared with age matched controls. LDL-C levels were also higher even in studies with BMI matching [8.32 mg/dl, 95% CI (5.82,10.81] [78].

The exact underlying mechanisms that involved to developing dyslipidemia in PCOS are not clearly described, but it has been hypothesized that the intertwined effects of obesity, insulin resistance and hyperandrogenism induce dyslipidemia among women with PCOS [79-81].

The mechanisms by which obesity is associated with dyslipidemia in women with PCOS include insulin resistance, overproduction of VLDL, abnormal lipoprotein lipase-mediated lipolysis and a defect in the insulin-signaling pathway mediated by an overexpression of PI3KR1 gene [81]. Androgens decrease catabolic removal of LDL by attenuating estrogen receptor-mediated induction of LDL receptor activity and also upregulate of genes responsible for catabolism of HDL [81, 82]. In addition, IR leads to hepatic overproduction of apolipoprotein B-containing VLDL and hypertriglyceridemia [81, 82]. In particular, IR increases the production of VLDL, decreases the elimination of VLDL and chylomicrons from the circulation and increases the clearance of apolipoprotein A, the major component of HDL-C [83, 84].

Those lipid metabolic dysfunction in women with PCOS definitely exaggerates the risk for cardiovascular disease (CVD) with aging [79].

Although various patterns of dyslipidemia have been described, the most common profile mong women with PCOS is generally characterized by increased serum concentration of low density lipoprotein cholesterol (LDL-C) and very-low density lipoprotein cholesterol (VLDL-C), triglyceride (TG) and free fatty acid, as well as decreased serum level of high density lipoprotein cholesterol (HDL-C), particularly HDL2-C, due to reduced apolipoprotein A-I (apoA-I) [59, 85] and higher level of oxidized LDL-C, independent of BMI, [86]. However, this atherogenic profile is exacerbated by increased BMI and IR. However, the lipoprotein profile in PCOS is therefore similar to that seen in T2DM patients [51]. Therefore, it is worth noting that lipid pattern in women with PCOS is only modestly more atherogenic compared with healthy women with similar BMI [51].

However, there are some concerns that most of those available evidence usually derived from clinical-based studies with small sample sizes, lacked appropriate control groups, used heterogeneous diagnostic criteria, and did not adjust potential confounders. Moreover, clinical-based studies might be misleading; they present severe phenotypes of PCOS women referred for treatment. On the other hand, a population-based study might include younger, lower BMI women with less severe phenotypes that might have never been referred.

However, long-term population-based cohort study, did not confirmed the higher risk of dyslipidemia compared to general population [4].

However, population based studies with larger sample sizes and long term follow up are still recommended to show whether these risks reemerge later in life.

1.3.3. Hypertension

There are some evidence showed that blood pressure, particularly systolic blood pressure may increase in PCOS patients [51]. In this respect, Obesity and insulin resistance are considered key factors for the alteration of blood pressure in women with PCOS [87]. Insulin resistance and compensatory hyperinsulinemia in PCOS leads to an imbalance in the autonomic nervous system, increased renal sodium reabsorption, as well as a reduction in the production of nitric oxide [88, 89]. As well, it could interfere with the endothelium-dependent vasodilatation mechanisms causing vascular muscle wall hypertrophy [90, 91]. Obesity and central obesity as most prevalent feature in PCOS, lead to metabolic, endothelial and vascular dysfunction, neuroendocrine imbalances, sodium retention, glomerular hyperfiltration, proteinuria, and maladaptive immune and inflammatory responses; all associated with hypertension [92] among women with PCOS. Endothelial dysfunction is a major forerunner of obesity-related hypertension by impairing control of the vascular tone and by promoting structural changes of the vessel wall [61, 93]. Furthermore, renin-angiotensin system activation [94] due to hyperandrogenism and endothelial dysfunction due to increased endothelin-1 levels in women with PCOS regardless of BMI [87, 95] may play a role in developing of hypertension in the syndrome.

However, the studies addressing the prevalence of HTN in PCOS had conflicting results. Observational studies reported that the prevalence of hypertension, mainly systolic blood pressure in PCOS women is estimated at 9–25.7%, higher than the general population [96-99]. However, other cohort studies did not confirm a higher incidence of hypertension [4, 100]. A results of meta-analysis confirmed a greater risk of HTN in PCOS patients but demonstrates that this risk is increased only in reproductive age women with PCOS, indicating that after menopause, having a history of PCOS may not be as an important predisposing factor for developing HTN [101].

In conclusion, evidence about whether or not rates of hypertension increase differently over time in women with PCOS is inconclusive. There might be a predisposition of these women to hypertension in later life that may set the milieu for potential accelerated progression of cardiovascular events irrespective of BMI and centripetal obesity [102], the assumption need to be further clarified.

1.3.4. Obesity

Obesity is a key contributor to the clinical and metabolic manifestations of PCOS patients. However, there is little debate about the association between obesity, especially central obesity, and cardiovascular risk factors. Several methods are used to assess the content and distribution of body fat. BMI assessment is commonly used for evaluation of obesity and prediction of adverse cardio-metabolic outcomes as strong predictor for IR and metabolic syndrome [103]. Recently some metabolic parameters of lipids were added to adiposity indices for better prognostic evaluation of cardio-metabolic adverse events. However, less is known regarding the complex adiposity indexes, in women with PCOS. However, there are some studies showed that lipid accumulation product (LAP) [104], visceral adiposity index (VAI) [105] and a body shape index (ABSI) [103] were a good tool for assessing cardiometabolic risk in among PCOS patients.

In this respect, it is well recognized that a large proportion of women with PCOS are suffering from overweight, obesity and central obesity compared with age-matched controls [8, 18, 51, 103]. In a meta-analysis, women with PCOS had two fold higher risk of overweight (RR: 1.95; 95% CI:1.52, 2.50), three fold higher risk of obesity (RR: 2.77; 95% CI: 1.88, 4.10) and two fold central obesity (RR:1.73; 95% CI: 1.31, 2.30) compared to healthy women [106]. Although, magnetic resonance imaging (MRI) in women with PCOS and health controls matched for BMI and fat mass showed no difference in body fat distribution [107, 108], however, increased waist to hip ratio affects between 50-70% of those patients, independent to BMI [10, 109].

In general, Adipose tissue in PCOS is characterized by aberrant cellularity, which probably alters adipose tissue function and most likely contributes to metabolic disturbances in women with the syndrome. Adipocyte size reflects the balance between triglyceride storage and mobilization [110]. Overweight or obesity in PCOS may be attributable to IR, which leads to hyperinsulinemia that stimulates ovarian steroidogenesis and subsequent reduction in sex hormone-binding globulin (SHBG) [111]. Obesity could also increase the androgens, particularly total testosterone and free androgen index that can lead to the accumulation of visceral fat causing central obesity [80, 112]. In addition, obesity through obesity-related haemodynamic and metabolic abnormalities, leads to increased circulating blood volume, systemic vascular resistance, and activation of SNS and the renin-angiotensin system, that could potentially increase the risk of hypertension and CVD [113, 114]. Moreover, visceral obesity is associated with low-grade inflammation and raised inflammatory cytokines and proinflammatory factors such as TNF-α, interleukin-6 (IL-6) and interleukin-18 (IL-18), which are secreted by activated tissue marcophages infiltrated in adipose tissue, both of which are associated with CVD in patients with PCOS [115-117]. However, all of those alteration are related to metabolic and reproductive disturbances in PCOS patients and strongly influences the severity of its clinical, cardiometabolic, and endocrine disturbances in these women.

1.3.5. Adipokines

PCOS is closely associated with adipose tissue dysfunction [11]. Androgen excess, as experienced by women with PCOS, is often associated with adipocyte hypertrophy and both adipose tissue hypertrophy and hyperandrogenism are strongly associated with IR [11]. As well, Chronic low-grade inflammation in PCOS is also associated with androgen excess and to the hypertrophy of adipocytes, leading to adipose tissue dysfunction and altered secretion of cytokines [118].

Adipose tissue is an active endocrine organ and release a large number of bioactive peptides, involving in the regulation of energy homeostasis, reproduction, insulin action, lipid metabolism and systemic inflammation [119] that is generally called adipokines. Emerging evidence suggest that abnormal production, release or function of adipokines are one of the important underlying potential mechanisms associated with the increased risk of cardio-metabolic risk factors and IR in PCOS [11, 120-122]. The two main important and well-known of adipokines are adiponectin and leptin.

Adiponectin, as an anti-inflammatory cytokine, is exclusively produced by adipose tissue and plays a role in a variety of functions including the anti-inflammatory, anti-atherogenic mediator, and insulin-sensitizing effects [123]. This peptide, is adversely associated with the adipocyte mass and visceral adiposity [124, 125]. There are some evidence reporting that the serum level of adiponectin was significantly decreased in disorders with IR including obesity, metabolic syndrome, diabetes, and obesity-related cardiovascular diseases [123, 126-128].

In a meta-analysis, it is showed that women with PCOS had significantly lower adiponectin level compared to healthy counterparts regardless of the degree of obesity [123]. Obesity, as a prevalent manifestation of PCOS, can downregulate adiponectin through alterations in the expression of adiponectin receptors and reduces the adiponectin sensitivity. It leads to insulin resistance that in turn aggravates hyperinsulinemia in women with PCOS [129]. In addition, some adiponectin gene polymorphism is more expressed in PCOS, which may be related to the reduced secretion of adiponectin [130].

In contrast to adiponectin, leptin has a central and peripheral regulatory role in energy expenditure regulation, based on to the levels of energy stored as body fat [131]. As such, insulin indirectly regulates the secretion of leptin through its trophic effect on adipocytes by stimulates leptin gene expression [132, 133]. Leptin may also contribute to increased level of androgens by inducing steroidogenesis and inhibiting neuropeptide Y, which leads to increasing serum level of gonadotropin releasing hormone (GnRH) and lutenizing hormone (LH) [59, 134]. Moreover, increased serum level of leptin is associated with systemic inflammation, IR and high risk of atherosclerosis [135, 136]. In a meta-analysis involving 991 women with PCOS and 898 controls, it is revealed the higher leptin concentration in patients with PCOS compared to healthy women (standardized mean difference: 1.62, 95% CI: 1.01-2.23) and obesity exacerbated the increased level of leptin in PCOS patients [137].

However, the profile of most adipokines in PCOS is not still understood and the studies focusing the role on other adipokines are insufficient and controversial. However, exact underlying physiological and pathophysiological function of adipokines in the regulation of obesity and PCOS needs to study the dynamic interaction between adipokines and other potential pathways. In this respect, some adipokines such as adiponectin, leptin, omentin, resistin, irisin, apelin, vaspin, and visfatin are more dependent on obesity and insulin pathways [10, 11, 131, 133, 138-143] and some such as chemerin are more involved in low-grade inflammatory responses [141, 144], even some may participate in both pathways.

However, there is a long way a head to understand the role of adipokines in PCOS, which may act as a link between obesity and PCOS.

1.3.6. Metabolic Syndrome

Metabolic syndrome (MetS) is a cluster of endocrinopathy and metabolic disturbances including hyperglycemia/insulin resistance, central obesity, dyslipidemia and hypertension [145]. Among women, it is diagnosed by the presence of any three of the following criteria including (i) increased waist circumference of ≥ 90 cm, (ii) increased triglycerides of ≥ 150 mg/dL, (iii) decreased HDL-C of < 50 mg/dL, (iv) increased blood pressure including ≥ 130 mmHg for systolic and/or ≥ 85 mmHg for diastolic and (v) increased fasting glucose ≥ 100 mg/dL [146].

Women with PCOS potentially have an elevated risk of the individual components of MetS including dyslipidemia, hyperglycemia and hypertension [147-149]. These patients also have increased novel and nontraditional cardiovascular risk factors including elevated carotid intima media wall thickness and coronary artery calcification, increased inflammatory cytokines, endothelial dysfunction, arterial stiffness, carotid or aortic plaque [21, 111, 150-153]. It is suggested that IR in PCOS plays a major role in the pathway of potential pathological mechanisms responsible for the development of MetS in women with PCOS [111, 154, 155]. The potential underlying of clinical manifestations of MetS is debated in this chapter.

However, the results of studies about the risk of MetS in PCOS is controversial. In a meta-analysis, women with PCOS had a higher prevalence of MetS (OR 3.35, 95% CI 2.44, 4.59), particularly in overweight or obese PCOS patients (OR 1.88, 95% 1.16, 3.04) but not in lean women (OR 1.45, 95% CI 0.35, 6.12) [111]. In contrast, in another recent meta-analysis, the odds of MetS had no differences between adults with PCOS compared to healthy controls in population-based studies. These results were confirmed by the subgroup meta- analysis of some studies using age and BMI adjustment/matching [156], indicating that age, BMI and study design can affect the risk of MetS in PCOS.

1.4. PCOS and Non-Traditional Cardio-Metabolic Risk Factors

1.4.1. Hyperandrogenism and Severe PCOS Phenotypes

It is well documented that androgen excess as the most prominent feature in PCOS, *per se*, is also correlated with CVD in female [157]. Hyperandrogenism is closely associated with aggravation of central obesity, IR, atherogenic lipid profile including lowering HDL-C and increasing LDL-C [158, 159] which are the metabolic core for the development of CVD. Although obesity may play a role, but it is demonstrated that testosterone could increase angiotensinogen and renin gene expression which contribute to hypertension [160-162]. Moreover, it have been found to increase the appetite [163], chronic inflammation, and oxidative stress associated with PCOS [164-166]and also involve in anxious and depressed mood states [167, 168]. Along with metabolic effects, androgens directly have adverse effect on vasculature, promoting endothelial dysfunction [169-172] and accelerating atherosclerotic alterations [20, 173].

Women with severe phenotypes PCOS, mainly phenotype A and B who have, seems to have a more adverse cardio-metabolic profile, particularly increased prevalence of glucose intolerance and metabolic syndrome and also worse lipid profile with higher LDL and non-HDL cholesterols compared to milder phenotypes [78, 158, 174, 175]. However, it appear to be generally related to androgen excess, adiposity and central adiposity in those subPCOS population [158].

1.4.2. Chronic Inflammation

Evidence in support of the presence of chronic low-grade systemic inflammation a as a key contributor to the underlying pathogenesis of PCOS is incontrovertible. There is a genetic basis for the inflammation reported in PCOS [176]. It is demonstrated that women with PCOS have decreased anti-inflammatory agents, such as adiponectin and omentin [105], and increased proinflammatory cytokines such as C-reactive protein (CRP), TNF-α [177-179], interleukin-18, monocyte chemoattractant protein-1, oxidative stress and white blood count are increasing in women with PCOS [13, 179-181], independent of obesity and BMI, consistent with a chronic low-grade inflammatory state. However, chronic inflammation is strongly associated with development, progression, and prognosis of endothelial dysfunction and CV events in PCOS patients [179, 182]. As such, Inflammation is also likely to be associated with other prominent aspects of PCOS including insulin resistance and hyperandrogenism [180, 183]. However, further studies required to clear the role of inflammation in developing CVD in PCOS.

1.4.3. Oxidative Stress

Oxidants are chemical products that tend to gain electrons losing positive charge. They include products of normal cellular metabolism including reactive oxygen species (ROS) and reactive nitrogen species that derive from nitric oxide (RNS). ROS derive from molecular oxygen, and include oxygen ions, free radicals (chemical species with unpaired electrons) and peroxides [184]. Oxidative stress is characterized by as the imbalance between production and scavenging of oxidants and antioxidants [185]. Oxidants excess leads to DNA, cellular lipids and proteins damage, and could disturb their physiological function. Therefore, oxidative stress may involves in many underlying pathophysiology of human pathologic situation as well as in the physiologic process of ageing [186].

Emerging evidence revealed that oxidative circulating markers are significantly increased in patients with PCOS compared to healthy women [187]. In this respect, homocysteine, asymmetric dimethylarginine, and malondialdehyde as a promoters and by-products of oxidative stress are increased in women with PCOS, contrary, glutathione and paraoxonase-1 as antioxidants are decreased in women with PCOS independent of age and BMI [184, 188] which may shows that oxidative stress play an important role in pathophysiology of PCOS.

Obesity, androgen excess, insulin resistance and dyslipidemia in PCOS could induce inflammatory response oxidative stress by increased ROS-related oxidative stress, muscle activity to carry excessive weight, hyperleptinemia, chronic inflammation and inadequate antioxidant defences in PCOS, [189] even in the absence of excess adiposity [190)]. Circulating and molecular markers of oxidative stress and inflammation are also highly correlated with circulating androgens [116, 117]. Nevertheless, the effect of the abnormalities in oxidative stress is relatively small, and their clinical significance as cardiovascular risk factors needs to be precisely defined in future.

1.4.4. Haemostasis and Fibrinolysis Imbalance

There is no doubt that haemostatic system abnormalities could increase arterial and venous thromboembolism as important cardiovascular risk factors [191]. However, there is relatively strong literature suggesting that PCOS is associated with increased platelet aggregation and impaired plasma fibrinolytic activity with increased plasminogen activator inhibitor-1 and plasminogen [192, 193]. Those risks are exacerbated by oral contraceptive use, as a common PCOS treatment strategy [194]. Although those abnormalities are likely to increase cardiovascular disease in PCOS population, however further studies are warranted.

1.4.5. Vitamin D Deficiency

Vitamin D is a fat-soluble vitamin that is synthesized endogenously by sunlight-stimulated photochemical conversion of cholesterol to 7-dehydrocholesterol in the skin or obtained from the diet [195]. Vitamin D is known for its primary role in bone and mineral homeostasis. However recent evidence demonstrates its vitamin D deficiency contributes in a spectrum of pathologic process of metabolic disturbances and CVD [196]. Evidence has demonstrated that vitamin D receptor complex regulates genes contributed in glucose and lipid metabolism and also in blood pressure regulation, thereby indicating a role of vitamin D deficiency in the underlying pathogenesis of cardiovascular disease [197]. In this respect, vitamin D deficiency increases both insulin resistance and activation of proinflammatory process leading to glucose intolerance by β-cell damage and death. Moreover, it may activate the epigenetic alterations by hypermethylation in many diabetes-related genes as a feature of diabetes [198, 199]. It is showed that vitamin D deficiency has a negative effect on lipid profile particularly on total cholesterol and LDL cholesterol, apolipoprotein AI and HDL cholesterol levels [200, 201]. Moreover, Calcitriol is a pro-inflammatory and anti-inflammatory cellular cytokines modulator [202]. There is some evidence that vitamin D deficiency is negatively correlated with inflammatory markers such as CRP concentrations [203]. As well, Vitamin D also imply a crucial role in the modulation of innate and adaptive immune response in various inflammatory and autoimmune disorders. It is now recognized that active metabolite vitamin D receptors are expressed in cells of the immune system [204, 205].

However, vitamin D regulates about 3% of the human genome, including genes that are crucial for glucose and lipid metabolism, via its nucleoprotein receptor that binds to vitamin D response elements found in the promoter region of responsive genes [206].

However, studies showed that vitamin D deficiency are so prevalent among women with PCOS and it may play a key role in the development of PCOS [207, 208]. The genetic variant of the VDR was found to have an association with severity of clinical features of PCOS, but none with disease risk [206]. As well a recent meta-analysis showed that lower serum vitamin D levels were related to metabolic and hormonal disorders in women with PCOS, particularly dysglycemia including increased levels of fasting glucose and insulin resistance compared to those without vitamin D deficiency [209, 210]. However, result of studies focusing on the effect of vitamin D supplementation on metabolic and endocrine parameters in PCOS in insufficient and inconclusive. Therefore, given the heterogeneity of the current available studies, a definite conclusion is difficult to make. Well-designed randomized controlled trials are still needed to clarify the effect vitamin D deficiency treatment on cardio-metabolic disturbances in PCOS population.

1.5. PCOS and Cardiovascular Events

There is much more controversy regarding whether the risk of cardiovascular events are increased among women with PCOS [211, 212]. However, increased cardiovascular risk factors in PCOS is translated into increased risk for cardiovascular events remains to be established, considering that PCOS may improve with aging. In this respect, some studies have shown that hyperinsulinemia and hyperandrogenemia are independently associated with the presence of atherosclerosis and cardiovascular events [159, 213]. However, most probably, PCOS phenomenon and therefore the attributed cardiovascular risks in women with PCOS progressively normalizes with aging. It has been reported that the progressive reduction of ovarian and adrenal androgen secretion in the decade preceding menopause reduces the risk factors [214].

In agreement with this hypothesis, a recent published metanalysis evaluated the prevalence and hazard ratio of cardiovascular events among reproductive and menopausal women with PCOS, compared to healthy controls. However, 16 studies were included for final meta-analysis. Results showed that the pooled hazard of CV events in PCOS patients in both subgroups of reproductive and menopausal age were significantly 1.5 fold higher than healthy controls. However, sub group analysis among studies with population-based design, which may show the general PCOS population characteristics, revealed that the HR of CV events increased only in reproductive age PCOS patients, whereas the difference was not statistically significant when comparing menopausal PCOS patients to healthy controls [215]. It may suggested that history of PCOS during reproductive ages may not be a great risk factor for developing cardiovascular events in later life. At present, well designed, long term population based prospective studies, initiated in the reproductive period, are needed to clarify it.

CONCLUSION

PCOS is a common heterogeneous endocrinopathy among reproductive-aged women with significant adverse health impacts. Both traditional and non-traditional cardiometabolic risk factors may interact in PCOS, contributing to increased cardiometabolic risks, which are further exacerbated by high rates of concomitant obesity. Nevertheless, there is much more controversy regarding whether cardio-metabolic disease are increased in PCOS in later life, leaving many issues regarding cardiovascular and metabolic events unresolved. Overall, at present methodological heterogenicity, failure to control of confounders and also absence of long term follow up of PCOS population have hampered progress in understanding cardiometabolic aspects in PCOS. Larger-scale studies that address these gaps are needed to better characterize mechanisms and interrelationships between those factors that are intrinsic to PCOS.

REFERENCES

[1] Sirmans SM, Pate KA. Epidemiology, diagnosis, and management of polycystic ovary syndrome. *Clinical epidemiology.* 2014;6:1.

[2] Tehrani FR, Simbar M, Tohidi M, Hosseinpanah F, Azizi F. The prevalence of polycystic ovary syndrome in a community sample of Iranian population: Iranian PCOS prevalence study. *Reproductive Biology and Endocrinology.* 2011;9(1):39.

[3] Yildiz BO, Bozdag G, Yapici Z, Esinler I, Yarali H. Prevalence, phenotype and cardiometabolic risk of polycystic ovary syndrome under different diagnostic criteria. *Human reproduction.* 2012;27(10):3067-73.

[4] Behboudi-Gandevani S, Tehrani FR, Hosseinpanah F, Khalili D, Cheraghi L, Kazemijaliseh H, et al. Cardiometabolic risks in polycystic ovary syndrome: long-term population-based follow-up study. *Fertility and sterility.* 2018;110(7):1377-86.

[5] Escobar-Morreale HF. Polycystic ovary syndrome: definition, aetiology, diagnosis and treatment. *Nature Reviews Endocrinology.* 2018;14(5):270.

[6] de Melo AS, Dias SV, de Carvalho Cavalli R, Cardoso VC, Bettiol H, Barbieri MA, et al. Pathogenesis of polycystic ovary syndrome: multifactorial assessment from the foetal stage to menopause. *Reproduction.* 2015;150(1):R11-R24.

[7] Noroozzadeh M, Behboudi-Gandevani S, Zadeh-Vakili A, Tehrani FR. Hormone-induced rat model of polycystic ovary syndrome: A systematic review. *Life sciences.* 2017;191:259-72.

[8] Behboudi-Gandevani S, Ramezani Tehrani F, Rostami Dovom M, Farahmand M, Bahri Khomami M, Noroozzadeh M, et al. Insulin resistance in obesity and polycystic ovary syndrome: systematic review and meta-analysis of observational studies. *Gynecological Endocrinology.* 2016;32(5):343-53.

[9] Panidis D, Tziomalos K, Misichronis G, Papadakis E, Betsas G, Katsikis I, et al. Insulin resistance and endocrine characteristics of the different phenotypes of polycystic ovary syndrome: a prospective study. *Human reproduction.* 2012;27(2):541-9.

[10] Behboudi-Gandevani S, Tehrani FR, Yarandi RB, Noroozzadeh M, Hedayati M, Azizi F. The association between polycystic ovary syndrome, obesity, and the serum concentration of adipokines. *Journal of endocrinological investigation.* 2017;40(8):859-66.

[11] Spritzer PM, Lecke SB, Satler F, Morsch DM. Adipose tissue dysfunction, adipokines, and low-grade chronic inflammation in polycystic ovary syndrome. *Reproduction.* 2015;149(5):R219-R27.

[12] Villa J, Pratley RE. Adipose tissue dysfunction in polycystic ovary syndrome. *Current diabetes reports.* 2011;11(3):179.

[13] Duleba AJ, Dokras A. Is PCOS an inflammatory process? *Fertility and sterility.* 2012;97(1):7-12.

[14] Shorakae S, Teede H, de Courten B, Lambert G, Boyle J, Moran LJ, editors. *The emerging role of chronic low-grade inflammation in the pathophysiology of polycystic ovary syndrome. Seminars in reproductive medicine;* 2015: Thieme Medical Publishers.

[15] Hyderali BN, Mala K. Oxidative stress and cardiovascular complications in polycystic ovarian syndrome. *European Journal of Obstetrics & Gynecology and Reproductive Biology.* 2015;191:15-22.

[16] Papalou O, M Victor V, Diamanti-Kandarakis E. Oxidative stress in polycystic ovary syndrome. *Current pharmaceutical design.* 2016; 22(18):2709-22.

[17] Legro RS, editor. *Obesity and PCOS: implications for diagnosis and treatment. Seminars in reproductive medicine;* 2012: Thieme Medical Publishers.

[18] Lim S, Norman RJ, Davies M, Moran L. The effect of obesity on polycystic ovary syndrome: a systematic review and meta-analysis. *Obesity Reviews.* 2013;14(2):95-109.

[19] Allameh Z, Rouholamin S, Adibi A, Mehdipour M, Adeli M. Does carotid intima-media thickness have relationship with polycystic ovary syndrome? *International journal of preventive medicine.* 2013;4(11):1266.

[20] Meyer ML, Malek AM, Wild RA, Korytkowski MT, Talbott EO. Carotid artery intima-media thickness in polycystic ovary syndrome: a systematic review and meta-analysis. *Human reproduction update.* 2012;18(2):112-26.

[21] Calderon-Margalit R, Siscovick D, Merkin SS, Wang E, Daviglus ML, Schreiner PJ, et al. Prospective association of polycystic ovary syndrome with coronary artery calcification and carotid-intima-media thickness: the Coronary Artery Risk Development in Young Adults Women's study. *Arteriosclerosis, thrombosis, and vascular biology.* 2014;34(12):2688-94.

[22] Carmina E. Diagnosis of polycystic ovary syndrome: from NIH criteria to ESHRE-ASRM guidelines. *Minerva ginecologica.* 2004; 56(1):1-6.

[23] Azziz R, Carmina E, Dewailly D, Diamanti-Kandarakis E, Escobar-Morreale HF, Futterweit W, et al. The Androgen Excess and PCOS Society criteria for the polycystic ovary syndrome: the complete task force report. *Fertility and sterility.* 2009;91(2):456-88.

[24] Balen AH, Laven JS, Tan SL, Dewailly D. Ultrasound assessment of the polycystic ovary: international consensus definitions. *Human reproduction update.* 2003;9(6):505-14.

[25] Eshre TR, Group A-SPCW. Revised 2003 consensus on diagnostic criteria and long-term health risks related to polycystic ovary syndrome. *Fertility and sterility.* 2004;81(1):19-25.

[26] Azziz R, Kintziger K, Li R, Laven J, Morin-Papunen L, Merkin SS, et al. Recommendations for epidemiologic and phenotypic research in polycystic ovary syndrome: an androgen excess and PCOS society resource. *Human Reproduction.* 2019;34(11):2254-65.

[27] Moran C, Arriaga M, Rodriguez G, Moran S. Obesity differentially affects phenotypes of polycystic ovary syndrome. *International journal of endocrinology.* 2012;2012.

[28] Tehrani FR, Rashidi H, Khomami MB, Tohidi M, Azizi F. The prevalence of metabolic disorders in various phenotypes of polycystic ovary syndrome: a community based study in Southwest of Iran. *Reproductive biology and endocrinology.* 2014;12(1):89.

[29] Tziomalos K. Cardiovascular Risk in the Different Phenotypes of Polycystic Ovary Syndrome. *Current pharmaceutical design.* 2016; 22(36):5547-53.

[30] Ramezani Tehrani F, Amiri M. Polycystic Ovary Syndrome in Adolescents: Challenges in Diagnosis and Treatment. *International journal of endocrinology and metabolism.* 2019;17(3):e91554.

[31] Fauser BC, Tarlatzis BC, Rebar RW, Legro RS, Balen AH, Lobo R, et al. Consensus on women's health aspects of polycystic ovary syndrome (PCOS): the Amsterdam ESHRE/ASRM-Sponsored 3rd

PCOS Consensus Workshop Group. *Fertility and sterility.* 2012; 97(1):28-38. e25.

[32] Legro RS, Arslanian SA, Ehrmann DA, Hoeger KM, Murad MH, Pasquali R, et al. Diagnosis and treatment of polycystic ovary syndrome: an Endocrine Society clinical practice guideline. *The Journal of Clinical Endocrinology & Metabolism.* 2013; 98(12):4565-92.

[33] Noroozzadeh M, Tehrani FR, Sedaghat K, Godini A, Azizi F. The impact of prenatal exposure to a single dose of testosterone on insulin resistance, glucose tolerance and lipid profile of female rat's offspring in adulthood. *Journal of endocrinological investigation.* 2015; 38(5):489-95.

[34] Ajmal N, Khan SZ, Shaikh R. Polycystic ovary syndrome (PCOS) and genetic predisposition: A review article. *European journal of obstetrics & gynecology and reproductive biology:* X. 2019:100060.

[35] Panda PK, Rane R, Ravichandran R, Singh S, Panchal H. Genetics of PCOS: a systematic bioinformatics approach to unveil the proteins responsible for PCOS. *Genomics data.* 2016;8:52-60.

[36] Salehi Jahromi M, Hill JW, Ramezani Tehrani F, Zadeh-Vakili A. Hypomethylation of specific CpG sites in the promoter region of steroidogeneic genes (GATA6 and StAR) in prenatally androgenized rats. *Life sciences.* 2018;207:105-9.

[37] Salehi Jahromi M, Ramezani Tehrani F, Hill JW, Noroozzadeh M, Zarkesh M, Ghasemi A, et al. Alteration in follistatin gene expression detected in prenatally androgenized rats. *Gynecological endocrinology : The official journal of the International Society of Gynecological Endocrinology.* 2017;33(6):433-7.

[38] Zadeh-Vakili A, Ramezani Tehrani F, Daneshpour MS, Zarkesh M, Saadat N, Azizi F. Genetic polymorphism of vitamin D receptor gene affects the phenotype of PCOS. *Gene.* 2013;515(1):193-6.

[39] Escobar-Morreale HF, Luque-Ramírez M, San Millán JL. The molecular-genetic basis of functional hyperandrogenism and the polycystic ovary syndrome. *Endocrine reviews.* 2005;26(2):251-82.

[40] Prapas N, Karkanaki A, Prapas I, Kalogiannidis I, Katsikis I, Panidis D. Genetics of polycystic ovary syndrome. *Hippokratia*. 2009; 13(4):216.

[41] Diamanti-Kandarakis E, Kandarakis H, Legro RS. The role of genes and environment in the etiology of PCOS. *Endocrine*. 2006; 30(1):19-26.

[42] Merkin SS, Phy JL, Sites CK, Yang D. Environmental determinants of polycystic ovary syndrome. *Fertility and sterility*. 2016; 106(1):16-24.

[43] Zhang J, Liu X, Liu Y, Xu L, Zhou L, Tang L, et al. Environmental risk factors for women with polycystic ovary syndrome in china: a population-based case-control study. *Journal of biological regulators and homeostatic agents*. 2014;28(2):203-11.

[44] Longo S, Bollani L, Decembrino L, Di Comite A, Angelini M, Stronati M. Short-term and long-term sequelae in intrauterine growth retardation (IUGR). *The Journal of Maternal-Fetal & Neonatal Medicine*. 2013;26(3):222-5.

[45] Wells JC. The thrifty phenotype: an adaptation in growth or metabolism? *American Journal of Human Biology*. 2011;23(1):65-75.

[46] Escobar-Morreale HF, Álvarez-Blasco F, Botella-Carretero JI, Luque-Ramírez M. The striking similarities in the metabolic associations of female androgen excess and male androgen deficiency. *Human Reproduction*. 2014;29(10):2083-91.

[47] Hakim C, Padmanabhan V, Vyas AK. Gestational hyperandrogenism in developmental programming. *Endocrinology*. 2017;158(2):199-212.

[48] Gur EB, Karadeniz M, Turan GA. Fetal programming of polycystic ovary syndrome. *World journal of diabetes*. 2015;6(7):936.

[49] Noroozzadeh M, Tehrani FR, Khomami MB, Azizi F. A comparison of sexual function in women with polycystic ovary syndrome (PCOS) whose mothers had PCOS during their pregnancy period with those without PCOS. *Archives of sexual behavior*. 2017;46(7):2033-42.

[50] Cassar S, Misso ML, Hopkins WG, Shaw CS, Teede HJ, Stepto NK. Insulin resistance in polycystic ovary syndrome: a systematic review

and meta-analysis of euglycaemic–hyperinsulinaemic clamp studies. *Human reproduction.* 2016;31(11):2619-31.

[51] Randeva HS, Tan BK, Weickert MO, Lois K, Nestler JE, Sattar N, et al. Cardiometabolic aspects of the polycystic ovary syndrome. *Endocrine reviews.* 2012;33(5):812-41.

[52] Engmann L, Jin S, Sun F, Legro RS, Polotsky AJ, Hansen KR, et al. Racial and ethnic differences in the polycystic ovary syndrome metabolic phenotype. *American journal of obstetrics and gynecology.* 2017;216(5):493. e1-. e13.

[53] Jayagopal V, Kilpatrick E, Jennings P, Hepburn D, Atkin S. The biological variation of testosterone and sex hormone-binding globulin (SHBG) in polycystic ovarian syndrome: implications for SHBG as a surrogate marker of insulin resistance. *The Journal of Clinical Endocrinology & Metabolism.* 2003;88(4):1528-33.

[54] Luotola K, Piltonen TT, Puurunen J, Morin-Papunen LC, Tapanainen JS. Testosterone is associated with insulin resistance index independently of adiposity in women with polycystic ovary syndrome. *Gynecological Endocrinology.* 2018;34(1):40-4.

[55] Zhang B, Wang J, Shen S, Liu J, Sun J, Gu T, et al. Association of androgen excess with glucose intolerance in women with polycystic ovary syndrome. *BioMed research international.* 2018;2018.

[56] Diamanti-Kandarakis E, Panidis D. Unravelling the phenotypic map of polycystic ovary syndrome (PCOS): a prospective study of 634 women with PCOS. *Clinical endocrinology.* 2007;67(5):735-42.

[57] Paschou SA, Palioura E, Ioannidis D, Anagnostis P, Panagiotakou A, Loi V, et al. Adrenal hyperandrogenism does not deteriorate insulin resistance and lipid profile in women with PCOS. *Endocrine connections.* 2017;6(8):601-6.

[58] Tehrani FR, Zarkesh M, Tohidi M, Azizi F, Zadeh-Vakili A. Is the association between insulin resistance and diabetogenic haematopoietically expressed homeobox (HHEX) polymorphism (rs1111875) affected by polycystic ovary syndrome status? *Reproduction, fertility, and development.* 2017;29(4):670-8.

[59] Anagnostis P, Tarlatzis BC, Kauffman RP. Polycystic ovarian syndrome (PCOS): Long-term metabolic consequences. *Metabolism.* 2018;86:33-43.

[60] González F, Sia CL, Bearson DM, Blair HE. Hyperandrogenism induces a proinflammatory TNFα response to glucose ingestion in a receptor-dependent fashion. *The Journal of Clinical Endocrinology & Metabolism.* 2014;99(5):E848-E54.

[61] Luque-Ramírez M, Escobar-Morreale HF. Polycystic ovary syndrome as a paradigm for prehypertension, prediabetes, and preobesity. *Current hypertension reports.* 2014;16(12):500.

[62] Behboudi-Gandevani S, Abtahi H, Saadat N, Tohidi M, Tehrani FR. Effect of phlebotomy versus oral contraceptives containing cyproterone acetate on the clinical and biochemical parameters in women with polycystic ovary syndrome: a randomized controlled trial. *Journal of ovarian research.* 2019;12(1):78.

[63] Escobar-Morreale HF. Iron metabolism and the polycystic ovary syndrome. *Trends in Endocrinology & Metabolism.* 2012;23(10):509-15.

[64] Diamanti-Kandarakis E, Dunaif A. Insulin resistance and the polycystic ovary syndrome revisited: an update on mechanisms and implications. *Endocrine reviews.* 2012;33(6):981-1030.

[65] Moro C, Pasarica M, Elkind-Hirsch K, Redman LM. Aerobic exercise training improves atrial natriuretic peptide and catecholamine-mediated lipolysis in obese women with polycystic ovary syndrome. *The Journal of Clinical Endocrinology & Metabolism.* 2009;94(7):2579-86.

[66] Potter LR, Abbey-Hosch S, Dickey DM. Natriuretic peptides, their receptors, and cyclic guanosine monophosphate-dependent signaling functions. *Endocrine reviews.* 2006;27(1):47-72.

[67] Pivovarova O. Gogebakan O Kloting N Sparwasser A Weickert MO Haddad I Nikiforova VJ Bergmann A Kruse M Seltmann AC. Insulin up-regulates natriuretic peptide clearance receptor expression in the subcutaneous fat depot in obese subjects: a missing link between CVD

risk and obesity. *Journal of Clinical Endocrinology and Metabolism.* 2012;97:E731-E9.

[68] Frøssing S, Nylander M, Kistorp C, Skouby SO, Faber J. Effect of liraglutide on atrial natriuretic peptide, adrenomedullin, and copeptin in PCOS. *Endocrine connections.* 2018;7(1):115-23.

[69] Pereira VM, Honorato-Sampaio K, Martins AS, Reis FM, Reis AM. Downregulation of natriuretic peptide system and increased steroidogenesis in rat polycystic ovary. *Peptides.* 2014;60:80-5.

[70] Jaliseh HK, Tehrani FR, Behboudi-Gandevani S, Hosseinpanah F, Khalili D, Cheraghi L, et al. Polycystic ovary syndrome is a risk factor for diabetes and prediabetes in middle-aged but not elderly women: a long-term population-based follow-up study. *Fertility and sterility.* 2017;108(6):1078-84.

[71] Vrbikova J, Cifkova R, Jirkovska A, Lanska V, Platilova H, Zamrazil V, et al. Cardiovascular risk factors in young Czech females with polycystic ovary syndrome. *Human Reproduction.* 2003;18(5):980-4.

[72] Moran LJ, Misso ML, Wild RA, Norman RJ. Impaired glucose tolerance, type 2 diabetes and metabolic syndrome in polycystic ovary syndrome: a systematic review and meta-analysis. *Human reproduction update.* 2010;16(4):347-63.

[73] Kakoly N, Khomami M, Joham A, Cooray S, Misso M, Norman R, et al. Ethnicity, obesity and the prevalence of impaired glucose tolerance and type 2 diabetes in PCOS: a systematic review and meta-regression. *Human reproduction update.* 2018;24(4):455-67.

[74] Legro RS, Kunselman AR, Dodson WC, Dunaif A. Prevalence and predictors of risk for type 2 diabetes mellitus and impaired glucose tolerance in polycystic ovary syndrome: a prospective, controlled study in 254 affected women. *The journal of clinical endocrinology & metabolism.* 1999;84(1):165-9.

[75] Kakoly NS, Earnest A, Teede HJ, Moran LJ, Joham AE. The impact of obesity on the incidence of type 2 diabetes among women with polycystic ovary syndrome. *Diabetes care.* 2019;42(4):560-7.

[76] Conway G, Dewailly D, Diamanti-Kandarakis E, Escobar-Morreale HF, Franks S, Gambineri A, et al. The polycystic ovary syndrome: a

position statement from the European Society of Endocrinology. *European Journal of Endocrinology*. 2014;171(4):P1-P29.

[77] Yilmaz M, Biri A, Bukan N, Karakoç A, Sancak B, Törüner F, et al. Levels of lipoprotein and homocysteine in non-obese and obese patients with polycystic ovary syndrome. *Gynecological endocrinology*. 2005;20(5):258-63.

[78] Wild RA, Rizzo M, Clifton S, Carmina E. Lipid levels in polycystic ovary syndrome: systematic review and meta-analysis. *Fertility and sterility*. 2011;95(3):1073-9. e11.

[79] Wild RA. Dyslipidemia in PCOS. *Steroids*. 2012;77(4):295-9.

[80] Osibogun O, Ogunmoroti O, Michos ED. *Polycystic ovary syndrome and cardiometabolic risk: Opportunities for cardiovascular disease prevention*. Trends in cardiovascular medicine. 2019.

[81] Diamanti-Kandarakis E, Papavassiliou AG, Kandarakis SA, Chrousos GP. Pathophysiology and types of dyslipidemia in PCOS. *Trends in Endocrinology & Metabolism*. 2007;18(7):280-5.

[82] Macut D, Bjekić-Macut J, Savić-Radojević A. Dyslipidemia and oxidative stress in PCOS. *Polycystic Ovary Syndrome*. 40: Karger Publishers; 2013. p. 51-63.

[83] Sidhwani S, Scoccia B, Sunghay S, Stephens-Archer CN, Mazzone T, Sam S. Polycystic ovary syndrome is associated with atherogenic changes in lipoprotein particle number and size independent of body weight. *Clinical endocrinology*. 2011;75(1):76-82.

[84] Savage DB, Petersen KF, Shulman GI. Disordered lipid metabolism and the pathogenesis of insulin resistance. *Physiological reviews*. 2007;87(2):507-20.

[85] Hoffman LK, Ehrmann DA. Cardiometabolic features of polycystic ovary syndrome. *Nature clinical practice Endocrinology & metabolism*. 2008;4(4):215-22.

[86] Macut D, Damjanovic S, Panidis D, Spanos N, Glišić B, Petakov M, et al. Oxidised low-density lipoprotein concentration–early marker of an altered lipid metabolism in young women with PCOS. *European Journal of Endocrinology*. 2006;155(1):131-6.

[87] Macut D, Mladenović V, Bjekić-Macut J, Livadas S, Stanojlović O, Hrnčić D, et al. Hypertension in polycystic ovary syndrome: Novel insights. *Current hypertension reviews.* 2020;16(1):55-60.

[88] Marchesan LB, Spritzer PM. ACC/AHA 2017 definition of high blood pressure: implications for women with polycystic ovary syndrome. *Fertility and sterility.* 2019;111(3):579-87. e1.

[89] Marchesan LB, Spritzer PM. *Blood pressure: implications for women with polycystic ovary syndrome.* 2019.

[90] Zhou M-S, Wang A, Yu H. Link between insulin resistance and hypertension: What is the evidence from evolutionary biology? *Diabetology & metabolic syndrome.* 2014;6(1):12.

[91] Cascella T, Palomba S, Tauchmanovà L, Manguso F, Di Biase S, Labella D, et al. Serum aldosterone concentration and cardiovascular risk in women with polycystic ovarian syndrome. *The Journal of Clinical Endocrinology & Metabolism.* 2006;91(11):4395-400.

[92] DeMarco VG, Aroor AR, Sowers JR. The pathophysiology of hypertension in patients with obesity. *Nature Reviews Endocrinology.* 2014;10(6):364.

[93] Sprung V, Cuthbertson D, Pugh C, Daousi C, Atkinson G, Aziz N, et al. Nitric oxide-mediated cutaneous microvascular function is impaired in polycystic ovary sydrome but can be improved by exercise training. *The Journal of physiology.* 2013;591(6):1475-87.

[94] Alphan Z, Berberoglu Z, Gorar S, Candan Z, Aktas A, Aral Y, et al. Increased total Renin levels but not Angiotensin-converting enzyme activity in obese patients with polycystic ovary syndrome. *Medical Principles and Practice.* 2013;22(5):475-9.

[95] Diamanti-Kandarakis E, Spina G, Kouli C, Migdalis I. Increased endothelin-1 levels in women with polycystic ovary syndrome and the beneficial effect of metformin therapy. *The Journal of Clinical Endocrinology & Metabolism.* 2001;86(10):4666-73.

[96] Shi Y, Cui Y, Sun X, Ma G, Ma Z, Gao Q, et al. Hypertension in women with polycystic ovary syndrome: prevalence and associated cardiovascular risk factors. *European Journal of Obstetrics & Gynecology and Reproductive Biology.* 2014;173:66-70.

[97] Elting M, Korsen T, Bezemer P, Schoemaker J. Prevalence of diabetes mellitus, hypertension and cardiac complaints in a follow-up study of a Dutch PCOS population. *Human Reproduction.* 2001;16(3):556-60.

[98] Orbetzova M, Shigarminova R, Genchev G, Milcheva B, Lozanov L, Genov N, et al. Role of 24-hour monitoring in assessing blood pressure changes in polycystic ovary syndrome. *Folia medica.* 2003;45(3):21-5.

[99] Holte J, Gennarelli G, Berne C, Bergh T, Lithell H. Elevated ambulatory day-time blood pressure in women with polycystic ovary syndrome: a sign of a pre-hypertensive state? *Human reproduction.* 1996;11(1):23-8.

[100] Wild S, Pierpoint T, McKeigue P, Jacobs H. Cardiovascular disease in women with polycystic ovary syndrome at long-term follow-up: a retrospective cohort study. *Clinical endocrinology.* 2000;52(5):595-600.

[101] Amiri M, Ramezani Tehrani F, Behboudi-Gandevani S, Razieh B-Y, Carmina E. Risk of hypertension in women with polycystic ovary syndrome: a systematic review, meta-analysis and meta-regression. *Reproductive Biology and Endocrinology.* 2020;in press.

[102] Glueck CJ, Morrison JA, Goldenberg N, Wang P. Coronary heart disease risk factors in adult premenopausal white women with polycystic ovary syndrome compared with a healthy female population. *Metabolism.* 2009;58(5):714-21.

[103] Behboudi-Gandevani S, Tehrani FR, Cheraghi L, Azizi F. Could "a body shape index" and "waist to height ratio" predict insulin resistance and metabolic syndrome in polycystic ovary syndrome? *European Journal of Obstetrics & Gynecology and Reproductive Biology.* 2016;205:110-4.

[104] Wehr E, Gruber H-J, Giuliani A, Möller R, Pieber TR, Obermayer-Pietsch B. The lipid accumulation product is associated with impaired glucose tolerance in PCOS women. *The Journal of Clinical Endocrinology & Metabolism.* 2011;96(6):E986-E90.

[105] Agrawal H, Aggarwal K, Jain A. Visceral adiposity index: Simple Tool for assessing cardiometabolic risk in women with polycystic

ovary syndrome. *Indian journal of endocrinology and metabolism.* 2019;23(2):232.

[106] Lim SS, Davies M, Norman RJ, Moran L. Overweight, obesity and central obesity in women with polycystic ovary syndrome: a systematic review and meta-analysis. *Human reproduction update.* 2012;18(6):618-37.

[107] Manneräs-Holm L, Leonhardt H, Kullberg J, Jennische E, Odén A, Holm G, et al. Adipose tissue has aberrant morphology and function in PCOS: enlarged adipocytes and low serum adiponectin, but not circulating sex steroids, are strongly associated with insulin resistance. *The Journal of Clinical Endocrinology & Metabolism.* 2011; 96(2): E304-E11.

[108] Barber TM, Golding SJ, Alvey C, Wass JA, Karpe F, Franks S, et al. Global adiposity rather than abnormal regional fat distribution characterizes women with polycystic ovary syndrome. *The Journal of Clinical Endocrinology & Metabolism.* 2008;93(3):999-1004.

[109] Horejsi R, Möller R, Rackl S, Giuliani A, Freytag U, Crailsheim K, et al. Android subcutaneous adipose tissue topography in lean and obese women suffering from PCOS: comparison with type 2 diabetic women. *American Journal of Physical Anthropology: The Official Publication of the American Association of Physical Anthropologists.* 2004;124(3):275-81.

[110] Blouin K, Nadeau M, Perreault M, Veilleux A, Drolet R, Marceau P, et al. Effects of androgens on adipocyte differentiation and adipose tissue explant metabolism in men and women. *Clinical endocrinology.* 2010;72(2):176-88.

[111] Lim S, Kakoly N, Tan J, Fitzgerald G, Bahri Khomami M, Joham A, et al. Metabolic syndrome in polycystic ovary syndrome: a systematic review, meta-analysis and meta-regression. *Obesity reviews.* 2019; 20(2):339-52.

[112] Rachoń D, Teede H. Ovarian function and obesity—interrelationship, impact on women's reproductive lifespan and treatment options. *Molecular and cellular endocrinology.* 2010;316(2):172-9.

[113] Rahmouni K, Correia ML, Haynes WG, Mark AL. Obesity-associated hypertension: new insights into mechanisms. *Hypertension.* 2005; 45(1):9-14.

[114] Artham SM, Lavie CJ, Milani RV, Ventura HO. Obesity and hypertension, heart failure, and coronary heart disease—risk factor, paradox, and recommendations for weight loss. *Ochsner Journal.* 2009;9(3):124-32.

[115] Sathyapalan T, Atkin SL. Mediators of inflammation in polycystic ovary syndrome in relation to adiposity. *Mediators of inflammation.* 2010;2010.

[116] Lumeng CN, Saltiel AR. Inflammatory links between obesity and metabolic disease. *The Journal of clinical investigation.* 2011; 121(6):2111-7.

[117] Bañuls C, Rovira-Llopis S, de Marañon AM, Veses S, Jover A, Gomez M, et al. Metabolic syndrome enhances endoplasmic reticulum, oxidative stress and leukocyte–endothelium interactions in PCOS. *Metabolism.* 2017;71:153-62.

[118] Schiffer L, Arlt W, O'Reilly MW. Understanding the role of androgen action in female adipose tissue. *Hyperandrogenism in Women.* 53: Karger Publishers; 2019. p. 33-49.

[119] Durmus U, Duran C, Ecirli S. Visceral adiposity index levels in overweight and/or obese, and non-obese patients with polycystic ovary syndrome and its relationship with metabolic and inflammatory parameters. *Journal of endocrinological investigation.* 2017;40(5): 487-97.

[120] K Dimitriadis G, Kyrou I, S Randeva H. Polycystic ovary syndrome as a proinflammatory state: The role of adipokines. *Current pharmaceutical design.* 2016;22(36):5535-46.

[121] Chen X, Jia X, Qiao J, Guan Y, Kang J. Adipokines in reproductive function: a link between obesity and polycystic ovary syndrome. *J Mol Endocrinol.* 2013;50(2):R21-37.

[122] Delitala AP, Capobianco G, Delitala G, Cherchi PL, Dessole S. Polycystic ovary syndrome, adipose tissue and metabolic syndrome. *Archives of gynecology and obstetrics.* 2017;296(3):405-19.

[123] Toulis KA, Goulis D, Farmakiotis D, Georgopoulos N, Katsikis I, Tarlatzis B, et al. Adiponectin levels in women with polycystic ovary syndrome: a systematic review and a meta-analysis. *Human reproduction update.* 2009;15(3):297-307.

[124] Groth SW. Adiponectin and polycystic ovary syndrome. *Biological research for nursing.* 2010;12(1):62-72.

[125] Mirza SS, Shafique K, Shaikh AR, Khan NA, Qureshi MA. Association between circulating adiponectin levels and polycystic ovarian syndrome. *Journal of ovarian research.* 2014;7(1):18.

[126] Fasshauer M, Paschke R, Stumvoll M. Adiponectin, obesity, and cardiovascular disease. *Biochimie.* 2004;86(11):779-84.

[127] Antoniades C, Antonopoulos A, Tousoulis D, Stefanadis C. Adiponectin: from obesity to cardiovascular disease. *Obesity reviews.* 2009;10(3):269-79.

[128] Lee S, Kwak H-B. Role of adiponectin in metabolic and cardiovascular disease. *Journal of exercise rehabilitation.* 2014; 10(2):54.

[129] Drolet R, Bélanger C, Fortier M, Huot C, Mailloux J, Légaré D, et al. Fat depot-specific impact of visceral obesity on adipocyte adiponectin release in women. *Obesity.* 2009;17(3):424-30.

[130] Xita N, Georgiou I, Chatzikyriakidou A, Vounatsou M, Papassotiriou G-P, Papassotiriou I, et al. Effect of adiponectin gene polymorphisms on circulating adiponectin and insulin resistance indexes in women with polycystic ovary syndrome. *Clinical chemistry.* 2005;51(2):416-23.

[131] Athyros VG, Tziomalos K, Karagiannis A, Anagnostis P, Mikhailidis DP. Should adipokines be considered in the choice of the treatment of obesity-related health problems? *Current drug targets.* 2010;11(1): 122-35.

[132] Mendonça H, Montenegro Junior R, Foss MC, Silva de Sá M, Ferriani RA. Positive correlation of serum leptin with estradiol levels in patients with polycystic ovary syndrome. *Brazilian journal of medical and biological research.* 2004;37(5):729-36.

[133] Polak K, Czyzyk A, Simoncini T, Meczekalski B. New markers of insulin resistance in polycystic ovary syndrome. *Journal of endocrinological investigation.* 2017;40(1):1-8.

[134] Veldhuis JD, Pincus S, Garcia-Rudaz M, Ropelato M, Escobar M, Barontini M. Disruption of the synchronous secretion of leptin, LH, and ovarian androgens in nonobese adolescents with the polycystic ovarian syndrome. *The Journal of Clinical Endocrinology & Metabolism.* 2001;86(8):3772-8.

[135] Freitas Lima LC, Braga VdA, do Socorro de França Silva M, Cruz JdC, Sousa Santos SH, de Oliveira Monteiro MM, et al. Adipokines, diabetes and atherosclerosis: an inflammatory association. *Frontiers in physiology.* 2015;6:304.

[136] Hou N, Luo JD. Leptin and cardiovascular diseases. *Clinical and Experimental Pharmacology and Physiology.* 2011;38(12):905-13.

[137] Zheng S-H, Du D-F, Li X-L. Leptin levels in women with polycystic ovary syndrome: a systematic review and a meta-analysis. *Reproductive sciences.* 2017;24(5):656-70.

[138] Seow KM, Juan CC, Wu LY, Hsu YP, Yang WM, Tsai YL, et al. Serum and adipocyte resistin in polycystic ovary syndrome with insulin resistance. *Human Reproduction.* 2004;19(1):48-53.

[139] Kim JJ, Choi YM, Hong MA, Kim MJ, Chae SJ, Kim SM, et al. Serum visfatin levels in non-obese women with polycystic ovary syndrome and matched controls. *Obstetrics & gynecology science.* 2018; 61(2):253-60.

[140] Sun X, Wu X, Zhou Y, Yu X, Zhang W. Evaluation of apelin and insulin resistance in patients with PCOS and therapeutic effect of drospirenone-ethinylestradiol plus metformin. *Medical science monitor: international medical journal of experimental and clinical research.* 2015;21:2547.

[141] Guvenc Y, Var A, Goker A, Kuscu NK. Assessment of serum chemerin, vaspin and omentin-1 levels in patients with polycystic ovary syndrome. *Journal of International Medical Research.* 2016; 44(4):796-805.

[142] Yang X, Quan X, Lan Y, Wei Q, Ye J, Yin X, et al. Serum chemerin level in women with PCOS and its relation with the risk of spontaneous abortion. *Gynecological Endocrinology.* 2018;34(10): 864-7.

[143] Emekci Ozay O, Ozay AC, Acar B, Cagliyan E, Seçil M, Küme T. Role of kisspeptin in polycystic ovary syndrome (PCOS). *Gynecological Endocrinology.* 2016;32(9):718-22.

[144] Kort DH, Kostolias A, Sullivan C, Lobo RA. Chemerin as a marker of body fat and insulin resistance in women with polycystic ovary syndrome. *Gynecological Endocrinology.* 2015;31(2):152-5.

[145] Huang PL. A comprehensive definition for metabolic syndrome. *Disease models & mechanisms.* 2009;2(5-6):231-7.

[146] Grundy SM, Cleeman JI, Daniels SR, Donato KA, Eckel RH, Franklin BA, et al. Diagnosis and management of the metabolic syndrome: an American Heart Association/National Heart, Lung, and Blood Institute scientific statement. *Circulation.* 2005;112(17):2735-52.

[147] Melo AS, Vieira CS, Romano LGM, Ferriani RA, Navarro PA. The frequency of metabolic syndrome is higher among PCOS Brazilian women with menstrual irregularity plus hyperandrogenism. *Reproductive Sciences.* 2011;18(12):1230-6.

[148] Techatraisak K, Wongmeerit K, Dangrat C, Wongwananuruk T, Indhavivadhana S. Measures of body adiposity and visceral adiposity index as predictors of metabolic syndrome among Thai women with PCOS. *Gynecological Endocrinology.* 2016;32(4):276-80.

[149] Zhang J, Fan P, Liu H, Bai H, Wang Y, Zhang F. Apolipoprotein AI and B levels, dyslipidemia and metabolic syndrome in south-west Chinese women with PCOS. *Human reproduction.* 2012;27(8):2484-93.

[150] Samy N, Hashim M, Sayed M, Said M. Clinical significance of inflammatory markers in polycystic ovary syndrome: their relationship to insulin resistance and body mass index. *Disease markers.* 2009;26(4):163-70.

[151] Macut D, Bačević M, Božić-Antić I, Bjekić-Macut J, Čivčić M, Erceg S, et al. Predictors of subclinical cardiovascular disease in women

with polycystic ovary syndrome: interrelationship of dyslipidemia and arterial blood pressure. *International journal of endocrinology.* 2015;2015.

[152] Meyer C, McGrath BP, Teede HJ. Overweight women with polycystic ovary syndrome have evidence of subclinical cardiovascular disease. *The Journal of Clinical Endocrinology & Metabolism.* 2005; 90(10):5711-6.

[153] Dokras A. Cardiovascular disease risk in women with PCOS. *Steroids.* 2013;78(8):773-6.

[154] Essah PA, Wickham EP, Nestler JE. The metabolic syndrome in polycystic ovary syndrome. *Clinical obstetrics and gynecology.* 2007;50(1):205-25.

[155] Amiri M, Tehrani FR, Bidhendi-Yarandi R, Behboudi-Gandevani S, Azizi F, Carmina E. Relationships between biochemical markers of hyperandrogenism and metabolic parameters in women with polycystic ovary syndrome: A systematic review and meta-analysis. *Hormone and Metabolic Research.* 2019;51(01):22-34.

[156] Behboudi-Gandevani S, Amiri M, Bidhendi Yarandi R, Noroozzadeh M, Farahmand M, Rostami Dovom M, et al. The risk of metabolic syndrome in polycystic ovary syndrome: A systematic review and meta-analysis. *Clinical endocrinology.* 2018;88(2):169-84.

[157] Macut D, Antić I, Bjekić-Macut J. Cardiovascular risk factors and events in women with androgen excess. *Journal of endocrinological investigation.* 2015;38(3):295-301.

[158] Chiu W-L, Boyle J, Vincent A, Teede H, Moran LJ. Cardiometabolic risks in polycystic ovary syndrome: non-traditional risk factors and the impact of obesity. *Neuroendocrinology.* 2017;104(4):412-24.

[159] Wu FC, von Eckardstein A. Androgens and coronary artery disease. *Endocrine reviews.* 2003;24(2):183-217.

[160] Chen M-J, Yang W-S, Yang J-H, Chen C-L, Ho H-N, Yang Y-S. Relationship between androgen levels and blood pressure in young women with polycystic ovary syndrome. *Hypertension.* 2007; 49(6):1442-7.

[161] Chen Y-F, Naftilan AJ, Oparil S. Androgen-dependent angiotensinogen and renin messenger RNA expression in hypertensive rats. *Hypertension.* 1992;19(5):456-63.

[162] Sulaiman MA, Al-Farsi YM, Al-Khaduri MM, Saleh J, Waly MI. Polycystic ovarian syndrome is linked to increased oxidative stress in Omani women. *International journal of women's health.* 2018; 10:763.

[163] Krug I, Giles S, Paganini C. Binge eating in patients with polycystic ovary syndrome: prevalence, causes, and management strategies. *Neuropsychiatric disease and treatment.* 2019;15:1273.

[164] Diamanti-Kandarakis E, Alexandraki K, Piperi C, Protogerou A, Katsikis I, Paterakis T, et al. Inflammatory and endothelial markers in women with polycystic ovary syndrome. *European journal of clinical investigation.* 2006;36(10):691-7.

[165] Diamanti-Kandarakis E, Paterakis T, Kandarakis HA. Indices of low-grade inflammation in polycystic ovary syndrome. *Annals of the New York Academy of Sciences.* 2006;1092(1):175-86.

[166] Fenkci V, Fenkci S, Yilmazer M, Serteser M. Decreased total antioxidant status and increased oxidative stress in women with polycystic ovary syndrome may contribute to the risk of cardiovascular disease. *Fertility and sterility.* 2003;80(1):123-7.

[167] Ekholm UB, Turkmen S, Hammarbäck S, Bäckström T. Sexuality and androgens in women with cyclical mood changes and pre-menstrual syndrome. *Acta obstetricia et gynecologica Scandinavica.* 2014; 93(3):248-55.

[168] Cooney LG, Lee I, Sammel MD, Dokras A. High prevalence of moderate and severe depressive and anxiety symptoms in polycystic ovary syndrome: a systematic review and meta-analysis. *Human Reproduction.* 2017;32(5):1075-91.

[169] Kravariti M, Naka KK, Kalantaridou SN, Kazakos N, Katsouras CS, Makrigiannakis A, et al. Predictors of endothelial dysfunction in young women with polycystic ovary syndrome. *The journal of clinical endocrinology & metabolism.* 2005;90(9):5088-95.

[170] Paradisi G, Steinberg HO, Hempfling A, Cronin J, Hook G, Shepard MK, et al. Polycystic ovary syndrome is associated with endothelial dysfunction. *Circulation.* 2001;103(10):1410-5.

[171] Lambert EA, Teede H, Sari CI, Jona E, Shorakae S, Woodington K, et al. Sympathetic activation and endothelial dysfunction in polycystic ovary syndrome are not explained by either obesity or insulin resistance. *Clinical endocrinology.* 2015;83(6):812-9.

[172] El-Kannishy G, Kamal S, Mousa A, Saleh O, El Badrawy A, Shokeir T. Endothelial function in young women with polycystic ovary syndrome (PCOS): Implications of body mass index (BMI) and insulin resistance. *Obesity research & clinical practice.* 2010; 4(1):e49-e56.

[173] Karoli R, Fatima J, Siddiqi Z, Vatsal P, Sultania AR, Maini S. Study of early atherosclerotic markers in women with polycystic ovary syndrome. *Indian journal of endocrinology and metabolism.* 2012;16(6):1004.

[174] Pehlivanov B, Orbetzova M. Characteristics of different phenotypes of polycystic ovary syndrome in a Bulgarian population. *Gynecological endocrinology.* 2007;23(10):604-9.

[175] Hosseinpanah F, Barzin M, Keihani S, Ramezani Tehrani F, Azizi F. Metabolic aspects of different phenotypes of polycystic ovary syndrome: Iranian PCOS Prevalence Study. *Clinical endocrinology.* 2014;81(1):93-9.

[176] Escobar-Morreale HF, Botella-Carretero JI, Alvarez-Blasco F, Sancho J, San Millán JL. The polycystic ovary syndrome associated with morbid obesity may resolve after weight loss induced by bariatric surgery. *The Journal of Clinical Endocrinology & Metabolism.* 2005;90(12):6364-9.

[177] Erdogan M, Karadeniz M, Berdeli A, Alper G, Caglayan O, Yilmaz C. *The relationship of the interleukin-6-174 G> C gene polymorphism with oxidative stress markers in Turkish polycystic ovary syndrome patients.* Journal of endocrinological investigation. 2008;31(7):624-9.

[178] Möhlig M, Spranger J, Osterhoff M, Ristow M, Pfeiffer A, Schill T, et al. *CLINICAL STUDY: The polycystic ovary syndrome per se is not associated with increased chronic inflammation.* 2004.
[179] Escobar-Morreale HF, Luque-Ramírez M, González F. Circulating inflammatory markers in polycystic ovary syndrome: a systematic review and metaanalysis. *Fertility and sterility.* 2011;95(3):1048-58.e2.
[180] González F. Inflammation in polycystic ovary syndrome: underpinning of insulin resistance and ovarian dysfunction. *Steroids.* 2012;77(4):300-5.
[181] Blumenfeld Z. *The Possible Practical Implication of High CRP Levels in PCOS.* SAGE Publications Sage UK: London, England; 2019.
[182] Paquissi FC. The role of inflammation in cardiovascular diseases: the predictive value of neutrophil–lymphocyte ratio as a marker in peripheral arterial disease. *Therapeutics and clinical risk management.* 2016;12:851.
[183] Shorakae S, Ranasinha S, Abell S, Lambert G, Lambert E, de Courten B, et al. Inter-related effects of insulin resistance, hyperandrogenism, sympathetic dysfunction and chronic inflamma-tion in PCOS. *Clinical endocrinology.* 2018;89(5):628-33.
[184] Murri M, Luque-Ramírez M, Insenser M, Ojeda-Ojeda M, Escobar-Morreale HF. Circulating markers of oxidative stress and polycystic ovary syndrome (PCOS): a systematic review and meta-analysis. *Human reproduction update.* 2013;19(3):268-88.
[185] Pisoschi AM, Pop A. The role of antioxidants in the chemistry of oxidative stress: A review. *European journal of medicinal chemistry.* 2015;97:55-74.
[186] Valko M, Leibfritz D, Moncol J, Cronin MT, Mazur M, Telser J. Free radicals and antioxidants in normal physiological functions and human disease. *The international journal of biochemistry & cell biology.* 2007;39(1):44-84.
[187] Mohammadi M. Oxidative stress and polycystic ovary syndrome: A brief review. *International journal of preventive medicine.* 2019;10.

[188] Turrens JF. Mitochondrial formation of reactive oxygen species. *The Journal of physiology.* 2003;552(2):335-44.

[189] Vincent HK, Taylor AG. Biomarkers and potential mechanisms of obesity-induced oxidant stress in humans. *International journal of obesity.* 2006;30(3):400-18.

[190] González F, Rote NS, Minium J, Kirwan JP. Reactive oxygen species-induced oxidative stress in the development of insulin resistance and hyperandrogenism in polycystic ovary syndrome. *The Journal of Clinical Endocrinology & Metabolism.* 2006;91(1):336-40.

[191] Alexander CJ, Tangchitnob EP, Lepor NE. Polycystic ovary syndrome: a major unrecognized cardiovascular risk factor in women. *Reviews in Obstetrics and Gynecology.* 2009;2(4):232.

[192] Targher G, Zoppini G, Bonora E, Moghetti P, editors. Hemostatic and fibrinolytic abnormalities in polycystic ovary syndrome. *Seminars in thrombosis and hemostasis;* 2014: Thieme Medical Publishers.

[193] Nave AH, Lange KS, Leonards CO, Siegerink B, Doehner W, Landmesser U, et al. Lipoprotein (a) as a risk factor for ischemic stroke: a meta-analysis. *Atherosclerosis.* 2015;242(2):496-503.

[194] Burchall GF, Piva TJ, Linden MD, Gibson-Helm ME, Ranasinha S, Teede HJ, editors. Comprehensive assessment of the hemostatic system in polycystic ovarian syndrome. *Seminars in thrombosis and hemostasis;* 2016: Thieme Medical Publishers.

[195] Krul-Poel Y, Koenders P, Steegers-Theunissen R, Ten Boekel E, ter Wee M, Louwers Y, et al. Vitamin D and metabolic disturbances in polycystic ovary syndrome (PCOS): A cross-sectional study. *PloS one.* 2018;13(12).

[196] Rahimi-Ardabili H, Gargari BP, Farzadi L. Effects of vitamin D on cardiovascular disease risk factors in polycystic ovary syndrome women with vitamin D deficiency. *Journal of endocrinological investigation.* 2013;36(1):28-32.

[197] Bouillon R, Carmeliet G, Verlinden L, van Etten E, Verstuyf A, Luderer HF, et al. Vitamin D and human health: lessons from vitamin D receptor null mice. *Endocrine reviews.* 2008;29(6):726-76.

[198] Berridge MJ. Vitamin D deficiency and diabetes. *Biochemical Journal*. 2017;474(8):1321-32.
[199] Hu Z, Jin'an Chen XS, Wang L, Wang A. Efficacy of vitamin D supplementation on glycemic control in type 2 diabetes patients: a meta-analysis of interventional studies. *Medicine*. 2019;98(14).
[200] Pérez-López FR. Vitamin D metabolism and cardiovascular risk factors in postmenopausal women. *Maturitas*. 2009;62(3):248-62.
[201] Ge H, Sun H, Wang T, Liu X, Li X, Yu F, et al. The association between serum 25-hydroxyvitamin D3 concentration and serum lipids in the rural population of China. *Lipids in health and disease*. 2017;16(1):215.
[202] Talmor-Barkan Y, Bernheim J, Green J, Benchetrit S, Rashid G. Calcitriol counteracts endothelial cell pro-inflammatory processes in a chronic kidney disease-like environment. *The Journal of steroid biochemistry and molecular biology*. 2011;124(1-2):19-24.
[203] Liu W, Zhang L, Xu H-J, Li Y, Hu C-M, Yang J-Y, et al. The anti-inflammatory effects of vitamin D in tumorigenesis. *International journal of molecular sciences*. 2018;19(9):2736.
[204] Tiosano D, Wildbaum G, Gepstein V, Verbitsky O, Weisman Y, Karin N, et al. The Role of vitamin D receptor in innate and adaptive immunity: a study in hereditary vitamin D–resistant rickets patients. *The Journal of Clinical Endocrinology & Metabolism*. 2013; 98(4):1685-93.
[205] Hewison M. Vitamin D and immune function: an overview. *Proceedings of the Nutrition Society*. 2012;71(1):50-61.
[206] Zadeh-Vakili A, Tehrani FR, Daneshpour MS, Zarkesh M, Saadat N, Azizi F. Genetic polymorphism of vitamin D receptor gene affects the phenotype of PCOS. *Gene*. 2013;515(1):193-6.
[207] Mogili KD, Karuppusami R, Thomas S, Chandy A, Kamath MS, Aleyamma T. Prevalence of vitamin D deficiency in infertile women with polycystic ovarian syndrome and its association with metabolic syndrome–A prospective observational study. *European Journal of Obstetrics & Gynecology and Reproductive Biology*. 2018;229:15-9.

[208] Kensara OA. Prevalence of hypovitaminosis D, and its association with hypoadiponectinemia and hyperfollistatinemia, in Saudi women with naïve polycystic ovary syndrome. *Journal of clinical & translational endocrinology.* 2018;12:20-5.

[209] He C, Lin Z, Robb SW, Ezeamama AE. Serum vitamin D levels and polycystic ovary syndrome: a systematic review and meta-analysis. *Nutrients.* 2015;7(6):4555-77.

[210] Davis EM, Peck JD, Hansen KR, Neas BR, Craig L. Associations between vitamin D levels and polycystic ovary syndrome phenotypes. *Minerva endocrinologica.* 2019;44(2):176-84.

[211] Azziz R. Does the risk of diabetes and heart disease in women with polycystic ovary syndrome lessen with age? *Fertility and sterility.* 2017;108(6):959-60.

[212] Talbott EO, Zborowski JV, Sutton-Tyrrell K, McHugh-Pemu KP, Guzick DS. Cardiovascular risk in women with polycystic ovary syndrome. *Obstetrics and gynecology clinics of North America.* 2001;28(1):111-33.

[213] Mcfarlane SI, Banerji M, Sowers JR. Insulin resistance and cardiovascular disease. *The Journal of Clinical Endocrinology & Metabolism.* 2001;86(2):713-8.

[214] Carmina E, Campagna A, Lobo R. Emergence of ovulatory cycles with aging in women with polycystic ovary syndrome (PCOS) alters the trajectory of cardiovascular and metabolic risk factors. *Human Reproduction.* 2013;28(8):2245-52.

[215] Ramezani Tehrani F, Amiri M, Behboudi-Gandevani S, Bidhendi-Yarandi R, Carmina E. Cardiovascular events among reproductive and menopausal age women with polycystic ovary syndrome: a systematic review and meta-analysis. *Gynecological Endocrinology.* 2020; 36(1):12-23.

In: Cardiometabolic Diseases and Risk Factors   ISBN: 978-1-53618-111-1
Editor: Patrick Ralston   © 2020 Nova Science Publishers, Inc.

Chapter 3

CARDIOMETABOLIC RISKS RELATED TO OBESITY: POTENTIAL EFFECTS OF NUTRITIONAL HABITS

Danielle Cristina Seiva[1,2],
Yasmin Alaby Martins Ferreira[1,2],
Marcos Mônico-Neto[1,2,3],
Hanna Karen Moreira Antunes[1,2,3]
and Raquel Munhoz da Silveira Campos[1,2]

[1]Post Graduated Program of Interdisciplinary Health Sciences;
[2]Biosciences Department; Post Graduated Program of Psychobiology[3];
Universidade Federal de São Paulo – UNIFESP, Brazil

ABSTRACT

Obesity is considerate a global epidemic with alarming consequences. Epidemiology data indicate that approximately 2.1 billion of adult population has obesity diagnosis. Data from World Health Organization demonstrated that 36.20% in the United States, 27.80% in the United

Kingdom and 22.10% in Brazil adult population were obese. Obesity is a multifactorial disease related to increase of body fat mass, metabolic disorders and a pro-inflammatory state. This framework induces to development of many comorbidities, including dyslipidemia, metabolic syndrome, non-alcoholic fatty liver disease and increase the cardiovascular risk factors. Considering the cardiovascular diseases (CDVs), it represents the number 1 cause of death in the world. Mostly of the CVDs can be prevented by lifestyle changes, for example, increase the physical activity and improve the nutritional habits. Specially for diet habits, this is an area who has aroused a relevant interesting, since nutritional behavior is an important strategy to prevent and treat several diseases. In fact, the impact of nutrition habits in obesity and CVDs was expensively studied. Although, recently the pro/anti-inflammatory effects of diet aroused interest from the scientific community, suggesting that foods can exert influence in metabolism pathway and be able to contribute or prevent the disease development, as obesity and cardiovascular diseases. In this way, the dietary inflammatory score was development to characterize the pro/anti-inflammatory effects of individuals diet and permitted to explore the possible associations with metabolic alterations related to several disease. In this sense, the present chapter will be exploring the aspects of nutritional habits and diet quality in the mechanism associated to increase on cardiovascular risk factors in obese population.

OBESITY, INFLAMMATION AND CARDIOVASCULAR RISK

Obesity is considerate a global epidemic defined as an increase in body weight with an excessive accumulation of adipose tissue related to the development of several metabolic disorders resulting in many comorbidities as non-alcoholic fatty liver disease, metabolic syndrome, sleep disorders and cardiovascular diseases (Karczewski et al., 2018).

Countless factors have been recognized to involve in the etiology of obesity, including positive energy balance, intestinal dysbiosis, hormonal signal, demographics conditions, emotional behavior, sedentarism, inappropriate diet, metabolic, and endocrine alterations. It is relevant to note that the influence of related factors is highly variable, and most of the time, these factors are associated and never in isolation condition (Karczewski et al., 2018; Ghosh & Bouchard, 2017).

Epidemiology data showed that more than 1.9 billion of global adults were estimated to be overweight (body mass index ≥25 kg/m²), and approximately 650 million were obese (BMI ≥ 30 kg/m²) (WHO, 2017). It was reported that obesity affection has tripled in the last ten years, killing approximately 28 million people each year (Ortega-Loubon et al., 2019).

In addition, a higher prevalence of obesity is observed in women compared to men. In this context, it was related that some factors could contribute to the mortality and morbidity risk association with an increase of body mass index, such as, sedentary behaviors, an increase in visceral fat accumulation, smoking, increased age, and inappropriate quality diet. Indeed, it is plausible to reinforce that adopting a healthy lifestyle can reduce this relative risk associated with increased BMI (González-Muniesa et al., 2017).

A relevant fact linking obesity and comorbidities, especially cardiovascular diseases, is the different fat accumulation localization. Several investigations showed that visceral fat is considered the most deleterious adipose tissue function (Ragino et al., 2020; Hiuge-Shimizu et al., 2012; Andersson et al., 2011; Davis, 2011). Adipocytes localized in this area present higher β1 adrenergic receptors on the cell surface compared to subcutaneous adipocytes. Since, more lipolytic effects of catecholamines and a reduce anti-lipolytic of insulin were observed, which leads to greater mobilization of free fatty acids by lipolysis from visceral fatty deposits than subcutaneous deposits. In addition, in visceral fat occur a greater predominance of macrophages M1, involved in the production of pro-inflammatory markers as leptin, TNF-α, interleukin-6, PAI-1 and resistin (González-Muniesa et al., 2016). Moreover, the deposit of epicardial fat is related to increase of cardiovascular risk, characterized by higher levels of fatty acid uptake and fatty acid release due to lipolysis; epicardial fat secretes several adipokines and vasoactive substances that impact the adjacent myocardium, which is clinically related to comorbidities development (Chait & den Hartigh, 2020; Mazurek et al., 2003).

It is plausible to relate that expansion of adiposity tissue involves changes in lipid accumulation with a dynamic variation, associate especially with the variations in energy balance, for example, positive energy balance will resulting in a lipogenic activity, since every energy derives of diet (considering mainly a diet with higher ingest of lipids and carbohydrates) will be accumulated inside the adipocyte as triglycerides, and this process contributes to the adipose tissue expansion. The increase of adipocytes occurs by different mechanisms, through an increase in adipocyte size (hypertrophy) and adipocyte number (hyperplasia) (Tandon et al., 2018).

In this sense, the revision published by Klöting & Blüher (2014) demonstrated that endogenous and exogenous factors could contribute to the adipose tissue expansion, individuals that present an increase in size and number of adipocytes, hypertrophy, and hyperplasia, respectively, probably will demonstrate a normal adipose tissue function. However, individuals with an expansion of adipose tissue associated only with the increase in volume (adipocyte hypertrophy) are frequently associated with pathogenic factors, for example, an increase in pro-inflammatory adipokines secretion.

Thus, one of the most metabolic complications related in obesity condition is the presence of low-grade chronic inflammatory state defined as an increase of pro-inflammatory and reduction of anti-inflammatory adipocytokines, that is believed to be the most critical condition that contributes to the development of obesity comorbidities (Lumeng & Saltiel, 2011). Adipose tissue is considered an endocrine organ that secretes various substances and metabolites, as free fatty acids and adipokines. In obesity, the expansion of adipose tissue is related to an increase of pro-inflammatory adipokines production and contributes to the development of many metabolic disorders (Bouyanfif et al., 2019).

It is known that several adipocytokines are involved to the development of cardiovascular complications in obese individuals, as for example, 1) Leptin: involved in the progression of atherosclerosis, vascular inflammation, platelet aggregation, and thrombus formation, increase blood pressure, migration and proliferation of smooth muscle cells in arteries and related to arteries calcification. 2) Interleukin 6: increase hepatic secretion of C reactive protein (CRP), the influx of fatty free acid, and adhesin molecules VCAM-1 and ICAM-1. 3) Plasminogen Activator Inhibitor-1 (PAI-1): contribute to the atheroma plaques formation by increase the platelets and fibrin deposition, and 4) Tumor Necrosis factor-α (TNF-α):

related to stimulating the migration and conversion of monocytes to macrophages, favoring the apoptosis process in endothelial cells (Lovren et al., 2015; Campos et al., 2014; Anfossi et al., 2010).

On the other hand, adiponectin, the most anti-inflammatory adipokine, secrete by adipose tissue, can stimulate the production of nitric oxide, mitigation of pro-atherogenic mediators, coronary plaque stabilization, arterial vasodilation, protective factors that are resulting in a decrease of cardiovascular risk. Although, it is important to reinforce that in obesity condition, the adiponectin level is reduced, but the weight loss contribute to improve adiponectin level and the inflammatory state (Cercato & Fonseca, 2019).

Not only the inflammatory state could contribute to cardiovascular disease in obese individuals, but disturbances in microbiota could also increase the lipopolysaccharide (LPS) release in the bloodstream and consequently activates toll-like receptor 4 (TLR4) involve in the pro-inflammatory pathway, and insulin resistance develops (Cercato & Fonseca, 2019; Saad et al., 2016).

Especially considering cardiovascular risk, the presence of glucose intolerance, high levels of total and low-density lipoprotein (LDL) cholesterol, low levels of high-density lipoprotein (HDL), high blood pressure and pro-inflammatory adipocytokines are the most common risk factors linking obesity to cardiovascular events (Funtikova et al., 2015). Also, obesity is associate with hemodynamics changes in cardiovascular system including an increase in blood volume, arterial pressure and stress in left ventricle wall; Moreover, in the cardiac structure, it is note hypertrophy of left and right ventricles; systolic and diastolic dysfunction is observed in the left ventricle with possible associations of right ventricle failure (Ortega-Loubon et al., 2019). The most common cardiovascular comorbidities related to obesity is atherosclerosis, a progressive disease associated with lipids accumulation, fibrous and inflammatory elements in the artery wall (;Steyers & Miller, 2014; Morange & Alessi, 2013) (Figure 1).

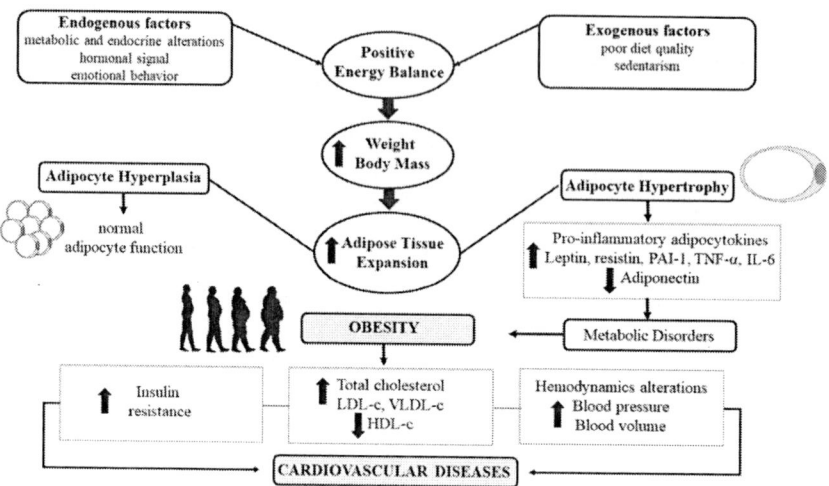

Figure 1. The obesity development is associate with a positive energy balance result of multifactorial components. The increase in weight body mass is related with expansion of adipose tissue by hyperplasia and hypertrophy of adipocytes. Adipocyte hypertrophy is associate with increase in several metabolic disorders, highlining the higher pro-inflammatory adipokines, such as leptin, plasminogen activator inhibitor type 1(PAI-1), Tumor necrosis factor-α (TNF- α), interleukin-6 (IL-6) and reduction in adiponectin level. In obesity, the presence of insulin resistance, alterations in lipid profile and hemodynamics complications contribute to increase the factors risks to develop cardiovascular diseases. Adaptation from Klöting & Blüher, 2014.

A diversity of interventions and strategies were explored to prevent and treat obesity and related comorbidities. In special, the incorporation of a healthy lifestyle, including regular physical exercise, sufficient hours of sleep, psychological and behavioral well-being, and dietary adequacy, are sources of benefits for the population in all age groups. Next, we will discuss the relevance of the nutritional factor in the development of obesity and cardiovascular risk in order to elucidate the benefits of a healthy diet.

DIETARY INFLAMMATORY INDEX, OBESITY AND CARDIOVASCULAR RISK

Dietary patterns play a role in the metabolism, glucose homeostasis, blood pressure and endothelial health that could culminate in obesity, inflammation by an excessive production of proinflammatory cytokines, and consequently cardiovascular disease, disability, and deaths (Mozaffarian, 2016; Minihane et al., 2015; Schwingshackl & Hoffmann G, 2014).

Current evidence pointed that Dietary Approaches to Stop Hypertension (DASH diet) and Mediterranean diet characterized by high fruits, vegetables, whole grains, low saturated fat, and low red meat intake had protective effects against cardiovascular disease and contributed to reducing inflammation and mortality (Chiavaroli et al., 2019; Ravera et al., 2016; Siervo et al., 2015; Sofi et al., 2014).

For each ingestion of 80 grams of fruits, it was associated with a decrease in 6-7% risk of coronary heart disease and cardiovascular disease in one UK Women's cohort study. Fruits and vegetables are rich in polyphenols and micronutrients that have anti-inflammatory and antioxidant activities, reducing oxidative stress and inflammation, protecting against atherosclerosis, and other cardiovascular diseases. Besides that, fruits and vegetables are a source of fibers (Serino & Salazar, 2019; Hosseini et al., 2018; Lai et al., 2015).

Dietary fiber has an important mechanism to decrease cholesterol levels and insulin secretion. Obesity and metabolic syndrome are frequently accompanied by insulin resistance. The triad of obesity, metabolic syndrome, and inflammation is characterized by cardiometabolic risk, which was negatively associated with dietary fiber intake. (Lie et al., 2018; Sima et al., 2018).

In addition to fiber and unsaturated fat, nuts have vitamin E, a fat-soluble vitamin that is involved in different pathways and have some efficacy in affect atherosclerotic plaque stability and reduce inflammation (Sozen et al., 2019; Ros, 2015).

Low consumption of vegetables, fruits, nuts, seeds, and omega-3 intake, and the excess of caloric intake, high processed meat was associated with cardiometabolic risk and deaths (Micha et al., 2017; Rocha et al., 2017; Schwandt et al., 2010).

The adult population in the world exceeds the recommended level of sodium intake, that are involved in increasing blood pressure, endothelial dysfunction, and modified renal functions. In 2010, one of ten deaths from cardiovascular outcomes were estimated by higher sodium intake globally. Individuals with obesity may benefit from reduced-sodium and adequate potassium intake in relation to cardiovascular health (Mozzafarian et al., 2014; Aaron & Sanders, 2013). The 2015-2020 Dietary Guidelines for Americans recommend consuming less than 2,300 milligrams per day of sodium (USDA, 2015).

The debate about health and dietary fat comes from decades. Substituting saturated fat with high glycemic index carbohydrates is associated with increased risk of cardiovascular diseases; however, dairy products that contain saturated fat and micronutrients such as Calcium and vitamin D may exert beneficial effects on obesity by ameliorating dyslipidemia, insulin resistance and blood pressure (Astrup, 2014).

A systematic review and meta-analysis of randomized controlled trials indicated that a low-fat diet had lower LDL-cholesterol, cholesterol, and HDL-c levels compared to high-fat diets. On the other hand, the excess of saturated fat and trans-fatty acid intake could alter blood lipid profile, increasing mainly LDL-cholesterol and triglycerides. Controversies results did not draw solid conclusions between dietary cholesterol and cardiovascular risk. Limit saturated fat in less than 10 percent per day of calories and replace it by unsaturated fat may be a strategy to improve serum lipoprotein profile and consequently reduce CVD risk (Carson et al., 2020; Forouhi et al., 2018; Lu et al., 2018; Mensink, 2016; Mozaffarian, 2016; USDA, 2015).

The interest in polyunsaturated fatty acids and cardiovascular disease increased since Bang & Dyerberg, 1972 investigated the plasma lipid and lipoprotein concentrations and Eskimos diet in Greenland compared to Danish people. The authors speculated that the low incidence of coronary atherosclerosis and diabetes mellitus in Eskimos are due to the low plasma lipid concentration and the composition of the diet (low content of saturated and high content of unsaturated fatty acids) (Bang et al., 1976; Bang & Dyeberg, 1972).

Omega-3, including eicosapentaenoic acid (EPA), docosahexaenoic acid (DHA), alpha-linolenic acid (ALA), are essential polyunsaturated fatty acids. The major source of ω-3 are marine organisms that contain EPA and

DHA; in addition, flax, chia, canola has ALA (Shahidi & Ambigaipalan, 2018). Modest lower risk of heart attacks is linked with blood biomarkers of seafood and plant-derived omega-3 fats. EPA and DHA intake and supplementation may be cardio-protective by decrease blood pressure, triglycerides, and contribute to regulate vascular function, exerting anti-inflammatory effects (Del Gobbo et al., 2016; Merino et al., 2014; Tousoulis et al., 2014; Calder, 2012; Wang et al., 2012).

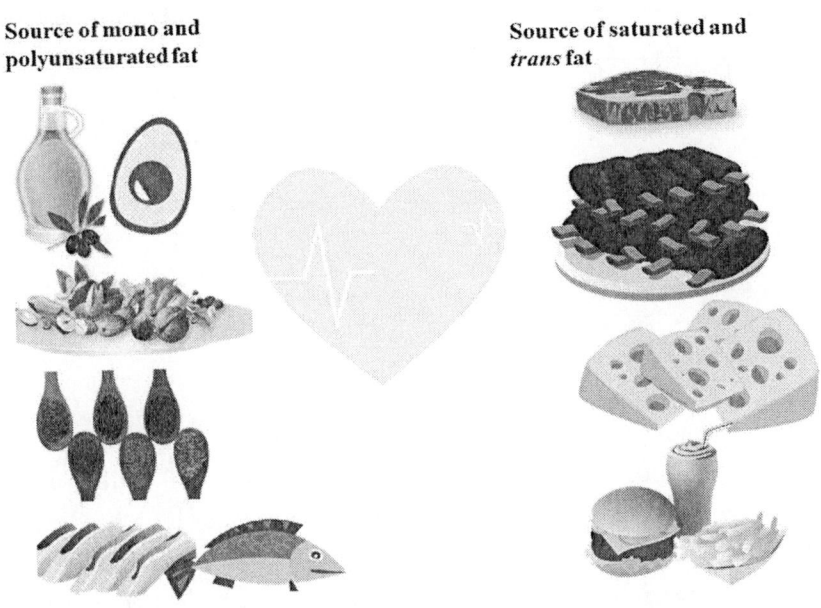

Figure 2. Fat intake could influence cardiovascular health. Foods that contain unsaturated fat are on the left side, while foods rich in saturated and *trans* fat are on the right side.

Abusive alcohol consumption is associated with heart attack and cardiovascular diseases. A recent study concluded that no dose of alcohol is safe to health (GBD, 2016). Some nutrients influence circulating concentrations of inflammatory markers, in view of this different index have been developed to assess the quality of diet and to associate it with non-communicable diseases and inflammation (Schwingshackl et al., 2018; Calder et al., 2011; Fung et al., 2005).

Dietary Inflammatory Index (DII) is an index created based on an extensive review of the literature to assess the potential inflammatory diet. It links forty-five food parameters (Table 1) with inflammatory biomarkers, such as interleukins 1β (IL-1β), IL-4, IL-6, IL-10, TNF-α, and C-reactive protein (CRP) (Shivappa et al., 2014).

Table 1. Food parameters included in DII

Alcohol	Eugenol	Monounsaturated fat	Saturated fat	Vitamin E	Isoflavones
Vitamin B12	Total fat intake	Polyunsaturated fat	Selenium	Zinc	Pepper
Vitamin B6	Fiber	n-3 fatty acids	Thiamin	Green/black tea	Thyme/oregano
B-Carotene	Folic acid	n-6 fatty acids	*Trans* fat	Flavon-3-ol	Rosemary
Caffeine	Garlic	Onion	Turmeric	Flavones	
Carbo-hydrate	Ginger	Protein	Vitamin A	Flavonols	
Cholesterol	Iron	Riboflavin	Vitamin C	Flavanones	
Energy intake	Magnesium	Saffron	Vitamin D	Anthocyanidins	

Adaptation from Shivappa et al., 2014.

Ruiz-Canela and colleagues (2015) found a negative association between pro-inflammatory diet (higher values of DII) with the Mediterranean diet and healthy food in individuals at high cardiovascular risk from a multicenter study "PREDIMED" in Spain. The authors found a positive association between pro-inflammatory diet and waist circumference. In the same cohort, Garcia-Arellano and colleagues (2015) found an association between higher DII score and higher cardiovascular risk.

Ferreira and colleagues (2019) found impairment in cardiometabolic parameters in adolescents with obesity who increased a pro-inflammatory diet after interdisciplinary therapy. Others studies showed positive associations between pro-inflammatory diet, cardiovascular disease, such myocardial infarction and mortality in different populations (Okada et al., 2019; Park et al., 2018; Shivappa et al., 2018; Namazi et al., 2018; Zhong et al., 2017; Ruiz-Canela et al., 2016).

By the way, given the complexity of obesity and cardiovascular disease, isolated nutrients have limited effects, considering nutrients or food are rarely consumed in isolation, and many dietary components and patterns contribute to obesity, the overall diet and foods must be taken into accounts to relate cardiometabolic risk (Carson et al., 2020; Forouhi et al., 2018; Mozaffarian, 2016).

INTESTINAL MICROBIOTA

A large number of bacteria, viruses, fungi, and archaea, especially in the colon, inhabits the human gastrointestinal tract (GIT). This composition of microorganisms is called intestinal microbiota. The Intestinal microbiota has functions in the homeostasis of the host controlling the metabolism and energy capture of nutrients, modulation of the immune system, regulation of the intestinal barrier, in addition to assisting in the synthesis of vitamins and in the digestive process (Krajmalnik-Brown et al., 2012).

Microbiota is composed of five main phyla *Firmicutes, Bacteroidetes, Proteobacteria, Actinobacteria* e *Verrucomicrobia* (Walker et al., 2011). In a healthy intestine, 90% of phyla are *Firmicutes* and *Bacteroidetes*; however the ratio between these phyla varies from individual to individual (Krajmalnik-Brown et al., 2012), for example, the intestinal microbiota of a subject with obesity diagnosis is characterized by an increase in the phylum *Firmicutes* and a reduction in the phylum *Bacteroidetes* (Ley et al., 2006).

Specifically, when we refer to the interaction between obesity and the risk for cardiovascular diseases (CVD), obesity is mainly characterized by an increase in body mass associated with an increase in fat mass. In the face of this condition, there are physiological adaptations of the organism among them, the increase in blood volume that consequently elevates the action of the left ventricle increasing cardiac debt, which can cause hypertrophy of the cardiac muscle and ventricular enlargement (right and left) predisposing to heart failure (HF) (Lavie et al., 2014).

A study (Abdullah et al., 2011) conducted with 5036 participants showed that mortality risk for all causes, mainly for CVD, in patients with obesity, increased according to the number of years in which these subjects showed the obesity diagnosis regardless of their current BMI. For every two years of obesity, the risk of mortality by CVD increases by 7% (Abdullah et al., 2011).

It is known that intestinal microbiota seems to perform an essential role in the interaction between obesity and CVD. However, to better understand the mechanisms involved, it is necessary to understand some previous concepts. It is known that in digestion, the intestinal microbiota is involved in two catabolic pathways. *Saccharolytic* pathway broke sugars and produces most short-chain fatty acids (SFCA), that are sources of energy for the intestinal epithelium, such as acetate, propionate, and butyrate (Lin et al., 2012) and proteolytic pathway, where the fermentation of proteins occurs forming metabolites like ammonia, thiols, indoles, phenols and amines (Gibson et al., 1989).

Intestinal microbiota synthesizes SFCA, especially for fermentation of polysaccharides and nondigested carbohydrates, in the proximal colon (Krajmalnik-Brown et al., 2012). Dietary energy uptake occurs when an SCFA binds to the protein G receptor, GPR41 (FFAR3), stimulating expression Peptide YY (PYY) in intestinal epithelial cells (Tazoe et al., 2009; Lin et al., 2012). Acetate and propionate are produced by phylum Bacteroidetes, where propionate seems to be produced by specie *Akkermansia muciniphila* (Morrison e Preston, 2016). The acetate is a substrate for lipogenesis *de novo* in the hepatocytes and adipocytes, and it is the precursor of cholesterol synthesis. While, propionate, stimulates gluconeogenesis in the hepatocytes (Krajmalnik-Brown et al., 2012).

Butyrate, produced by phylum *Firmicutes* (Louis et al., 2010) has the effect of suppressing the histone deacetylase, compromising chromatin structure interfering in nucleosomes (Henagan et al., 2015) and seems to possess an effect in the reduction of diastolic blood pressure by reducing inflammation (Roshanravan et al.; 2017). This SCFA also assists in maintaining the intestinal barrier by regulating protein complex (tight junctions), which forms a functional and structural intestinal barrier assisting in intestinal permeability, against cytokines pro-inflammatory (Yan e Ajuwon, 2017; Al-Sadi et al., 2008). Animals with a diet of high intake of salt change intestinal microbiota inducing T helper (Th)17 cells and supplementation with *Lactobacillus murinus* reduces the appearance of hypertension by restoring the defense of intestine (Wilck et al., 2017).

Blood pressure (BP) regulation occurs by stimulating GPR41 and GPR43 (FFAR2) receptors. GPR41 and GPR43 are expressed mainly in immune system cells, intestine, and adipose tissue. GPR41 is also expressed in the vascular endothelium, where it regulates BP (Natarajan et al., 2016) through renin secretion (Pluznick et al., 2013). A study performed in hypertensive Wistar Kyoto rats showed which microbiota of these animals was characterized by increased ratio *Firmicutes/Bacteroidetes* that increased blood pressure (Yang et al., 2015). However, posttransplant of cecal microbiota of normotensives animals to hypertensive animals, not enough to normalize dysbiosis or reduce the systolic indicating that transplant is host-dependent. While cecal transplant of hypertensive rats to normotensive rats have immediate effect exacerbating systolic BP (Mell et al., 2015), this study also registered that *Veillonellaceae* and *Bacteroidetes* communities were elevated in hypertensive rats (Mell et al., 2015).

Intestinal microbiota also metabolizes secondary biliary acids. Primary biliary acids, chenodeoxycholic acid, and cholic acid are unconjugated by microbiota transforming in secondary bile acids, deoxycholic acid, and lithocholic acid that assist in the absorption of dietary fats and fat-soluble vitamins. Secondary biliary acids signal the G-protein-coupled receptor 1 (TGR5) and farnesoid X receptor (FXR). Thus, it can alter glucose metabolism through FXR and modulate systemic and or hepatic lipid metabolism (Hylemon et al., 2009).

It is suggested that intestine microbial communities are a source of bacteria presents in atherosclerotic plaques, once the same was observed bacterial DNA in both locals in the same individuals, as the intestine and oral cavity and this situation can leave the development of CVD (Koren et al., 2011; Ott et al., 2006). Still, in this context, high levels of *Collinsella* bacteria were observed to increase oxidative stress and reduction of *Roseburia* bacteria in subjects with atherosclerosis (Karlsson et al., 2012). This environment was associated with a greater risk of developing cardiac events. Corroborating, colonies of bacteria of the genus *Veillonella*,

Streptococcus, and *Chryseomonas* were found to be present in most atherosclerotic samples (Koren et al., 2011).

It was checked in an experimental study, that intake of the western diet, characterized by refined grains, dairy with high-fat content, red and processed meat, sugary drinks, desserts and candies (Fung et al., 2004 e 2001; Hu et al., 2000) be intimately associated with a higher risk for the development of cardiovascular events. It was able to promote the reduction of *Akkermansia muciniphila* bacteria in the intestinal microbiota. However, these same animals, when treated with *Akkermansia muciniphila*, showed a reduction in the formation of atheroma plaques, decreased serum lipopolysaccharides (LPSs), reduced intestinal permeability and reduced aortic and systemic inflammation, thus suggesting the beneficial effect of this bacteria (Li et al., 2016; Everard et al., 2013).

Still, in this context, have trimethylamine (TMA), an amine present in some nutrients of diet (choline, phosphatidylcholine, and L-carnitine) is produced by intestinal microbiota through TMA-lyase. TMA is oxidized in the liver by the enzyme flavin monooxygenase (FMO) in trimethylamine-N-oxide (TMAO), where the kidney does excretion. This is an of pathways by which intestinal microbiota interacts with the host (Bennett et al., 2013). High levels of TMAO in plasma can predict increased risk for CVD (Bennett et al., 2013; Wang et al., 2011). Corroborating with this finding, it was verified the positive correlation between TMAO, derived from choline, L-carnitine and betaine, with the size of the atherosclerotic plaque, while for fasting blood glucose, triglycerides (TG), lipoproteins and triglycerides hepatic did not present an association in stable cardiac patients (Wang et al., 2011). Maybe this atherogenic effect has an association with the decrease of reverse cholesterol transport (Koeth et al., 2013).

High levels of TMAO in blood also were associated with an increased risk of myocardial infarction, stroke, death, and adverse cardiovascular events (Senthong et al., 2016). Circulating TMAO also found an increase in heart failure patients by increasing bacterial translocation in intestine increasing endotoxins and oxidative stress, but this pathway still not unclear (Sandek et al., 2007). In model animals, TMAO changed signaling platelet calcium and resulted in a prothrombotic effect in vivo (Zhu et al., 2016).

A study made with omnivores and vegans/vegetarians showed distinction in the composition of the intestinal microbiota of both, revealing that microbiota of vegans/vegetarians was able to produce less quantity TMA and TMAO from carnitine (Koeth et al., 2013).

SFCAs activate glucagon-like peptide-1 (GLP-1) through GPR43, which is activated mainly by acetate, propionate, and butyrate. Regarding body composition, in mice with overexpressing, GPR43 was observed eutrophic composition even when offered a high-fat diet, indicating that GPR43 can stimulate energy expenditure in muscle and liver on how to reduce fat accumulation (Kimura et al., 2013). On the other hand, rats that showed GPR43 deficiency showed obesity. In the mice in treatment with antibiotics or germ-free, with and without GPR43 deficiency, was observed appropriate body composition, indicating that activation of the GPR43 is AGCC dependent and may prevent the accumulation of fat for modulating awareness adipose tissue as for insulin. Meanwhile, the GPR41 is activated by propionate and butyrate and improves insulin signaling by stimulating PYY and GLP-1 secretion (Kimura et al., 2013).

An important class of bioactive are polyphenols. These are metabolized by the intestinal microbiota and bring benefits to the host avoiding CVD and diabetes. The apple is a well-explored example of fruit rich in polyphenols type catechin, flavanols, and fibers (Masumoto et al., 2016). Black tea also exhibits catechins that are converted into the colon and prevent CVD by preventing platelet aggregation, reducing BP, and are considered anti-inflammatory and anticoagulant (Khan and Mukhtar, 2007).

In fact, we know that food is able to modulate intestinal microbiota reducing CVD risk. According to the World Health Organization (WHO), healthy eating must have a low intake of saturated fats and adequate in sugars, salt, and fibers (WHO, 2019). It was observed in a study with human feces where 250mg of pea protein was incorporated, that glycated pea protein-maintained levels of SCFAs, and beneficially modulated the profile and metabolic activity of the microbiota (Świątecka et al., 2011).

Regarding fiber consumption, it was observed in an epidemiological study that was followed for 19 years, about 3700 cases of CVD incidents and 1800 cases of coronary heart disease (CHD) incidents, that people who consumed about 22g of fiber per day, particularly soluble, had 11% less risk of developing CVD and 12% less risk of developing CHD (Bazzano et al., 2003). Considering the fats, mice that were supplemented for 11 days with a diet based on lard (rich in saturated fat) increased the activation of Toll-like receptors (TLR), increasing inflammation of adipose tissue and decreasing insulin sensitivity. While mice supplemented with fish oil increased *Lactobacillus*, a probiotic associated with reducing inflammation and *Akkermansia muciniphila* associated with reduced macrophage infiltration and fat mass gain, in addition to improving glucose metabolism and intestinal barrier function (Caesar et al., 2015).

Finally, we have that composition of the diet can modulate the microbiota, as demonstrated in previous experimental and clinical studies, is considered a therapeutic strategy for CVD, although the mechanisms are still unknown. So, we understand that like obesity, metabolic syndrome, and diabetes mellitus, CVDs are also considered an important risk factor for reducing the increasing life expectancy more prevalent in recent years. An association of the intestinal microbiota with CVDs is increasingly being investigated, and it is known that it can contribute beneficially to the reduction of cardiovascular risk, promoting improvements in the health of the host. However, it is worth mentioning that this beneficial effect is conditioned to some factors that include lifestyle, body composition, and especially eating habits. In search of new knowledge and scientific development, omics sciences and metagenomic sequencing can assist in the investigation of better strategies in the microbiome together with the study of the participation at the molecular level of nutrients in cardiovascular diseases.

REFERENCES

Aaron KJ, Sanders PW. Role of dietary salt and potassium intake in cardiovascular health and disease: a review of the evidence. *Mayo Clin Proc.* 2013;88(9):987–995. doi:10.1016/j.mayocp.2013.06.005.

Abdullah A, Wolfe R, Stoelwinder JU, de Courten M, Stevenson C, Walls HL, Peeters A. The number of years lived with obesity and the risk of all-cause and cause-specific mortality. *Int J Epidemiol.* 2011 Aug;40(4):985-96. doi: 10.1093/ije/dyr018.

Al-Sadi R, Ye D, Dokladny K, Ma TY. Mechanism of IL-1beta-induced increase in intestinal epithelial tight junction permeability. *J Immunol.* 2008 Apr 15;180(8):5653-61. doi: 10.4049/jimmunol.180.8.5653.

Andersson DP, Löfgren P, Thorell A, Arner P, Hoffstedt J. Visceral fat cell lipolysis and cardiovascular risk factors in obesity. *Horm Metab Res.* 2011 Oct;43(11):809-15. doi: 10.1055/s-0031-1287767.

Anfossi G, Russo I, Doronzo G, Pomero A, Trovati M. Adipocytokines in atherothrombosis: focus on platelets and vascular smooth muscle cells. *Mediators Inflamm.* 2010; 2010:174341. doi: 10.1155/2010/174341.

Astrup A. Yogurt and dairy product consumption to prevent cardiometabolic diseases: epidemiologic and experimental studies. *Am J Clin Nutr.* 2014; 99(5 Suppl):1235S–42S. doi:10.3945/ajcn.113.073015.

Bang HO, Dyerberg J, Hjøorne N. The composition of food consumed by Greenland Eskimos. *Acta Med Scand.* 1976; 200(1-2):69–73. doi: 10.1111/j.0954-6820.1976.tb08198.x.

Bang HO, Dyerberg J. Plasma lipids and lipoproteins in Greenlandic west coast Eskimos. *Acta Med Scand.* 1972;192(1-2):85–94. doi: 10.1111/j.0954-6820.1972.tb04782.x.

Bazzano LA, He J, Ogden LG, Loria CM, Whelton PK; National Health and Nutrition Examination Survey I Epidemiologic Follow-up Study. Dietary fiber intake and reduced risk of coronary heart disease in US men and women: the National Health and Nutrition Examination Survey I Epidemiologic Follow-up Study. *Arch Intern Med.* 2003 Sep 8; 163(16):1897-904.

Bennett BJ, de Aguiar Vallim TQ, Wang Z, Shih DM, Meng Y, Gregory J, Allayee H, Lee R, Graham M, Crooke R, Edwards PA, Hazen SL, Lusis AJ. Trimethylamine-N-oxide, a metabolite associated with atherosclerosis, exhibits complex genetic and dietary regulation. *Cell Metab.* 2013 Jan 8;17(1):49-60. doi: 10.1016/j.cmet.2012.12.011.

Bouyanfif A, Jayarathne S, Koboziev I, Moustaid-Moussa N. The Nematode Caenorhabditis elegans as a Model Organism to Study Metabolic Effects of ω-3 Polyunsaturated Fatty Acids in Obesity. *Adv Nutr.* 2019 Jan 1;10(1):165-178. doi: 10.1093/advances/nmy059.

Caesar R, Tremaroli V, Kovatcheva-Datchary P, Cani PD, Bäckhed F. Crosstalk between Gut Microbiota and Dietary Lipids Aggravates WAT Inflammation through TLR Signaling. *Cell Metab.* 2015 Oct 6;22(4):658-68. doi: 10.1016/j.cmet.2015.07.026.

Calder PC, Ahluwalia N, Brouns F, et al. Dietary factors and low-grade inflammation in relation to overweight and obesity. *Br J Nutr.* 2011; 106 Suppl 3:S5–S78. doi: 10.1017/S0007114511005460.

Calder PC. Mechanisms of action of (n-3) fatty acids. *J Nutr.* 2012; 142(3):592S–599S. doi: 10.3945/jn.111.155259.

Campos RMS, Dâmaso AR, Masquio DCL. The impact of obesity on Carotid Artery Disease in Obese Adolescents Cap 4, 59-95. In: Derricks S. *Carotidy Artery Disease: risk factors, prognosis and management.* New York: Nova Medical, 2014.

Carson JAS, Lichtenstein AH, Anderson CAM, et al. Dietary Cholesterol and Cardiovascular Risk: A Science Advisory from the American Heart Association. *Circulation.* 2020;141(3):e39–e53. doi: 10.1161/CIR.0000000000000743.

Cercato C, Fonseca FA. Cardiovascular risk and obesity. *Diabetol Metab Syndr.* 2019 Aug 28;11:74. doi: 10.1186/s13098-019-0468-0.

Chait A, den Hartigh LJ. Adipose Tissue Distribution, Inflammation and Its Metabolic Consequences, Including Diabetes and Cardiovascular Disease. *Front Cardiovasc Med.* 2020 Feb 25;7:22. doi: 10.3389/fcvm.2020.00022.

Chiavaroli L, Viguiliouk E, Nishi SK, et al. DASH Dietary Pattern and Cardiometabolic Outcomes: An Umbrella Review of Systematic Reviews and Meta-Analyses. *Nutrients.* 2019;11(2):338. Published 2019 Feb 5. doi: 10.3390/nu11020338.

Davis S. Visceral fat accumulation and cardiovascular disease risk profile. *Climacteric.* 2011 Oct;14(5):599-600. PubMed PMID: 22016891.

Del Gobbo LC, Imamura F, Aslibekyan S, et al. ω-3 Polyunsaturated Fatty Acid Biomarkers and Coronary Heart Disease: Pooling Project of 19 Cohort Studies [published correction appears in JAMA Intern Med. 2016 Nov 1;176(11):1727-1728] [published correction appears in JAMA Intern Med. 2016 Nov 1;176(11):1728] [published correction appears in JAMA Intern Med. 2019 Mar 1;179(3):457]. *JAMA Intern Med.* 2016;176(8):1155–1166. doi: 10.1001/jamainternmed.2016.2925.

Everard A, Belzer C, Geurts L, Ouwerkerk JP, Druart C, Bindels LB, Guiot Y, Derrien M, Muccioli GG, Delzenne NM, de Vos WM, Cani PD. Cross-talk between Akkermansia muciniphila and intestinal epithelium controls diet-induced obesity. *Proc Natl Acad Sci U S A.* 2013 May 28;110(22):9066-71. doi: 10.1073/pnas.1219451110.

Ferreira YAM, Kravchychyn ACP, Vicente SCF, et al. An Interdiscipli-nary Weight Loss Program Improves Body Composition and Metabolic Profile in Adolescents With Obesity: Associations With the Dietary Inflammatory Index. *Front Nutr.* 2019;6:77. Published 2019 Jun 3. doi: 10.3389/fnut.2019.00077.

Forouhi NG, Krauss RM, Taubes G, Willett W. Dietary fat and cardiometabolic health: evidence, controversies, and consensus for guidance. *BMJ.* 2018 Jun 13;361:k2139. doi: 10.1136/bmj.k2139.

Fung TT, McCullough ML, Newby PK, et al. Diet-quality scores and plasma concentrations of markers of inflammation and endothelial dysfunction. *Am J Clin Nutr.* 2005; 82(1):163–173. doi: 10.1093/ajcn.82.1.163.

Fung TT, Rimm EB, Spiegelman D, Rifai N, Tofler GH, Willett WC, Hu FB. Association between dietary patterns and plasma biomarkers of obesity and cardiovascular disease risk. *Am J Clin Nutr.* 2001 Jan; 73(1):61-7.

Fung TT, Stampfer MJ, Manson JE, Rexrode KM, Willett WC, Hu FB. Prospective study of major dietary patterns and stroke risk in women. *Stroke.* 2004 Sep; 35(9):2014-9. Epub 2004 Jul 1.

Funtikova AN, Navarro E, Bawaked RA, Fíto M, Schröder H. Impact of diet on cardiometabolic health in children and adolescents. *Nutr J.* 2015 Nov 14;14:118. doi: 10.1186/s12937-015-0107-z.

Garcia-Arellano A, Ramallal R, Ruiz-Canela M, et al. Dietary Inflammatory Index and Incidence of Cardiovascular Disease in the PREDIMED Study. *Nutrients.* 2015;7(6):4124–4138. Published 2015 May 29. doi:10.3390/nu7064124.

GBD 2016 Alcohol Collaborators. Alcohol use and burden for 195 countries and territories, 1990-2016: a systematic analysis for the Global Burden of Disease Study 2016. *Lancet.* 2018 Sep 22;392(10152):1015-1035. doi: 10.1016/S0140-6736(18)31310-2.

Ghosh S, Bouchard C. Convergence between biological, behavioural and genetic determinants of obesity. *Nat Rev Genet.* 2017 Dec;18(12):731-748. doi: 10.1038/nrg.2017.72.

Gibson SA, McFarlan C, Hay S, MacFarlane GT. Significance of microflora in proteolysis in the colon. *Appl Environ Microbiol.* 1989 Mar; 55(3):679-83.

González-Muniesa P, Mártinez-González MA, Hu FB, Després JP, Matsuzawa Y, Loos RJF, Moreno LA, Bray GA, Martinez JA. Obesity. *Nat Rev Dis Primers.* 2017 Jun 15; 3:17034. doi: 10.1038/nrdp.2017.34.

Henagan TM, Stefanska B, Fang Z, Navard AM, Ye J, Lenard NR, Devarshi PP. Sodium butyrate epigenetically modulates high-fat diet-induced skeletal muscle mitochondrial adaptation, obesity and insulin resistance through nucleosome positioning. *Br J Pharmacol.* 2015 Jun; 172(11): 2782-98. doi: 10.1111/bph.13058.

Hiuge-Shimizu A, Kishida K, Funahashi T, Ishizaka Y, Oka R, Okada M, Suzuki S, Takaya N, Nakagawa T, Fukui T, Fukuda H, Watanabe N, Yoshizumi T, Ohira T, Nakamura T, Matsuzawa Y, Yamakado M, Shimomura I. Reduction of visceral fat correlates with the decrease in the number of obesity-related cardiovascular risk factors in Japanese with Abdominal Obesity (VACATION-J Study). *J Atheroscler Thromb.* 2012;19(11):1006-18.

Hosseini B, Berthon BS, Saedisomeolia A, et al. Effects of fruit and vegetable consumption on inflammatory biomarkers and immune cell populations: a systematic literature review and meta-analysis. *Am J Clin Nutr.* 2018;108(1):136–155. doi:10.1093/ajcn/nqy082.

Hu FB, Rimm EB, Stampfer MJ, Ascherio A, Spiegelman D, Willett WC. Prospective study of major dietary patterns and risk of coronary heart disease in men. *Am J Clin Nutr.* 2000 Oct;72(4):912-21.

Hylemon PB, Zhou H, Pandak WM, Ren S, Gil G, Dent P. Bile acids as regulatory molecules. *J Lipid Res.* 2009 Aug;50(8):1509-20. doi: 10.1194/jlr.R900007-JLR200.

Karczewski J, Śledzińska E, Baturo A, Jończyk I, Maleszko A, Samborski P, Begier-Krasińska B, Dobrowolska A. Obesity and inflammation. *Eur Cytokine Netw.* 2018 Sep 1;29(3):83-94. doi: 10.1684/ecn.2018.0415.

Karlsson FH, Fåk F, Nookaew I, Tremaroli V, Fagerberg B, Petranovic D, Bäckhed F, Nielsen J. Symptomatic atherosclerosis is associated with an altered gut metagenome. *Nat Commun.* 2012;3:1245. doi: 10.1038/ncomms2266.

Khan N, Mukhtar H. Tea polyphenols for health promotion. *Life Sci.* 2007 Jul 26;81(7):519-33. Epub 2007 Jun 28.

Kimura I, Ozawa K, Inoue D, Imamura T, Kimura K, Maeda T, TerasawaK, Kashihara D, Hirano K, Tani T, Takahashi T, Miyauchi S, Shioi G, Inoue H, Tsujimoto G. The gut microbiota suppresses insulin-mediated fat accumulation via the short-chain fatty acid receptor GPR43. *Nat Commun.* 2013;4:1829. doi: 10.1038/ncomms2852.

Klöting N, Blüher M. Adipocyte dysfunction, inflammation and metabolic syndrome. *Rev Endocr Metab Disord.* 2014 Dec;15(4):277-87. doi: 10.1007/s11154-014-9301-0.

Koeth RA, Wang Z, Levison BS, Buffa JA, Org E, Sheehy BT, Britt EB, Fu X, Wu Y, Li L, Smith JD, DiDonato JA, Chen J, Li H, Wu GD, Lewis JD, Warrier M, Brown JM, Krauss RM, Tang WH, Bushman FD, Lusis AJ, Hazen SL. Intestinal microbiota metabolism of L-carnitine, a nutrient in red meat, promotes atherosclerosis. *Nat Med.* 2013 May;19(5):576-85. doi: 10.1038/nm.3145.

Koren O, Spor A, Felin J, Fåk F, Stombaugh J, Tremaroli V, Behre CJ, Knight R, Fagerberg B, Ley RE, Bäckhed F. Human oral, gut, and plaque microbiota in patients with atherosclerosis. *Proc Natl Acad Sci U S A.* 2011 Mar 15;108 Suppl 1:4592-8. doi: 10.1073/pnas.1011383107.

Krajmalnik-Brown R, Ilhan ZE, Kang DW, DiBaise JK. Effects of gut microbes on nutrient absorption and energy regulation. *Nutr Clin Pract.* 2012 Apr;27(2):201-14. doi: 10.1177/0884533611436116.

Lai HT, Threapleton DE, Day AJ, Williamson G, Cade JE, Burley VJ. Fruit intake and cardiovascular disease mortality in the UK Women's Cohort Study. *Eur J Epidemiol.* 2015;30(9):1035–1048. doi: 10.1007/s10654-015-0050-5.

Lavie CJ, McAuley PA, Church TS, Milani RV, Blair SN. Obesity and cardiovascular diseases: implications regarding fitness, fatness, and severity in the obesity paradox. *J Am Coll Cardiol.* 2014 Apr 15;63(14):1345-54. doi: 10.1016/j.jacc.2014.01.022.

Ley RE, Turnbaugh PJ, Klein S, Gordon JI. Microbial ecology: human gut microbes associated with obesity. *Nature.* 2006 Dec 21;444(7122): 1022-3. P.

Li J, Lin S, Vanhoutte PM, Woo CW, Xu A. Akkermansia Muciniphila Protects Against Atherosclerosis by Preventing Metabolic Endotoxemia-Induced Inflammation in Apoe-/- Mice. *Circulation.* 2016 Jun 14;133(24):2434-46. doi: 10.1161/CIRCULATIONAHA.115.019645.

Lie L, Brown L, Forrester TE, et al. The Association of Dietary Fiber Intake with Cardiometabolic Risk in Four Countries across the Epidemiologic Transition. Nutrients. 2018;10(5):628. Published 2018 May 16. doi: 10.3390/nu10050628.

Lin HV, Frassetto A, Kowalik EJ Jr, Nawrocki AR, Lu MM, Kosinski JR, Hubert JA, Szeto D, Yao X, Forrest G, Marsh DJ. Butyrate and propionate protect against diet-induced obesity and regulate gut hormones via free fatty acid receptor 3-independent mechanisms. *PLoS One.* 2012;7(4):e35240. doi:10.1371/journal.pone.0035240.

Louis P, Young P, Holtrop G, Flint HJ. Diversity of human colonic butyrate-producing bacteria revealed by analysis of the butyryl-CoA:acetate CoA-transferase gene. *Environ Microbiol.* 2010 Feb;12(2):304-14. doi: 10.1111/j.1462-2920.2009.02066.x.

Lovren F, Teoh H, Verma S. Obesity and atherosclerosis: mechanistic insights. *Can J Cardiol.* 2015 Feb;31(2):177-83. doi: 10.1016/j.cjca.2014.11.031.

Lu M, Wan Y, Yang B, Huggins CE, Li D. Effects of low-fat compared with high-fat diet on cardiometabolic indicators in people with overweight and obesity without overt metabolic disturbance: a systematic review and meta-analysis of randomised controlled trials. *Br J Nutr.* 2018;119(1):96–108. doi: 10.1017/S0007114517002902.

Lumeng CN, Saltiel AR. Inflammatory links between obesity and metabolic disease. *J Clin Invest.* 2011 Jun;121(6):2111-7. doi: 10.1172/JCI57132.

Masumoto S, Terao A, Yamamoto Y, Mukai T, Miura T, Shoji T. Non-absorbable apple procyanidins prevent obesity associated with gut microbial and metabolomic changes. *Sci Rep.* 2016 Aug 10;6:31208. doi: 10.1038/srep31208.

Mazurek T, Zhang L, Zalewski A, Mannion JD, Diehl JT, Arafat H, Sarov-Blat L, O'Brien S, Keiper EA, Johnson AG, Martin J, Goldstein BJ, Shi Y. Human epicardial adipose tissue is a source of inflammatory mediators. *Circulation.* 2003 Nov 18;108(20):2460-6. Epub 2003 Oct 27.

Mell B, Jala VR, Mathew AV, Byun J, Waghulde H, Zhang Y, Haribabu B, Vijay-Kumar M, Pennathur S, Joe B. Evidence for a link between gut microbiota and hypertension in the Dahl rat. *Physiol Genomics.* 2015 Jun;47(6):187-97. doi: 10.1152/physiolgenomics.00136.2014.

Mensink, RP. *Effects of saturated fatty acids on serum lipids and lipoproteins: a systematic review and regression analysis.* Geneva: World Health Organization; 2016.

Merino J, Sala-Vila A, Kones R, et al. Increasing long-chain n-3PUFA consumption improves small peripheral artery function in patients at intermediate-high cardiovascular risk. *J Nutr Biochem.* 2014;25(6):642–646. doi:10.1016/j.jnutbio.2014.02.004.

Micha R, Peñalvo JL, Cudhea F, Imamura F, Rehm CD, Mozaffarian D. Association Between Dietary Factors and Mortality From Heart Disease, Stroke, and Type 2 Diabetes in the United States. *JAMA.* 2017 Mar 7;317(9):912-924. doi:10.1001/jama.2017.0947.

Minihane AM, Vinoy S, Russell WR, Baka A, Roche HM, Tuohy KM, Teeling JL, Blaak EE, Fenech M, Vauzour D, McArdle HJ, Kremer BH, Sterkman L, Vafeiadou K, Benedetti MM, Williams CM, Calder PC. Low-grade inflammation, diet composition and health: current research evidence and its translation. *Br J Nutr.* 2015 Oct 14;114(7):999-1012. doi: 10.1017/S0007114515002093.

Morange PE, Alessi MC. Thrombosis in central obesity and metabolic syndrome: mechanisms and epidemiology. *Thromb Haemost.* 2013 Oct;110(4):669-80. doi: 10.1160/TH13-01-0075.

Morrison DJ, Preston T. Formation of short chain fatty acids by the gut microbiota and their impact on human metabolism. *Gut Microbes.* 2016 May 3;7(3):189-200. doi: 10.1080/19490976.2015.1134082.

Mozaffarian D, Fahimi S, Singh GM, et al. Global sodium consumption and death from cardiovascular causes. *N Engl J Med.* 2014;371 (7):624–634. doi: 10.1056/NEJMoa1304127.

Mozaffarian D. Dietary and Policy Priorities for Cardiovascular Disease, Diabetes, and Obesity: A Comprehensive Review. *Circulation.* 2016 Jan 12;133(2):187-225. doi: 10.1161/CIRCULATIONAHA.115.018585.

Namazi N, Larijani B, Azadbakht L. Dietary Inflammatory Index and its Association with the Risk of Cardiovascular Diseases, Metabolic Syndrome, and Mortality: A Systematic Review and Meta-Analysis. *Horm Metab Res.* 2018;50(5):345–358. doi:10.1055/a-0596-8204.

Natarajan N, Hori D, Flavahan S, Steppan J, Flavahan NA, Berkowitz DE, Pluznick JL. Microbial short chain fatty acid metabolites lower blood pressure via endothelial G protein-coupled receptor 41. *Physiol Genomics.* 2016 Nov 1;48(11):826-834. doi: 10.1152/physiolgenomics. 00089.2016.

Okada E, Shirakawa T, Shivappa N, et al. Dietary Inflammatory Index Is Associated with Risk of All-Cause and Cardiovascular Disease Mortality but Not with Cancer Mortality in Middle-Aged and Older Japanese Adults. *J Nutr.* 2019;149(8):1451–1459. doi: 10.1093/jn/nxz085.

Ortega-Loubon C, Fernández-Molina M, Singh G, Correa R. Obesity and its cardiovascular effects. *Diabetes Metab Res Rev.* 2019 May; 35(4):e3135. doi: 10.1002/dmrr.3135.

Ott SJ, El Mokhtari NE, Musfeldt M, Hellmig S, Freitag S, Rehman A, Kühbacher T, Nikolaus S, Namsolleck P, Blaut M, Hampe J, Sahly H, Reinecke A, Haake N, Günther R, Krüger D, Lins M, Herrmann G, Fölsch UR, Simon R, Schreiber S. Detection of diverse bacterial signatures in atherosclerotic lesions of patients with coronary heart disease. *Circulation.* 2006 Feb 21;113(7):929-37.

Park SY, Kang M, Wilkens LR, et al. The Dietary Inflammatory Index and All-Cause, Cardiovascular Disease, and Cancer Mortality in the Multiethnic Cohort Study. *Nutrients.* 2018;10(12):1844. Published 2018 Dec 1. doi: 10.3390/nu10121844.

Pluznick JL, Protzko RJ, Gevorgyan H, Peterlin Z, Sipos A, Han J, Brunet I, Wan LX, Rey F, Wang T, Firestein SJ, Yanagisawa M, Gordon JI, Eichmann A, Peti-Peterdi J, Caplan MJ. Olfactory receptor responding to gut microbiota-derived signals plays a role in renin secretion and blood pressure regulation. *Proc Natl Acad Sci U S A.* 2013 Mar 12; 110(11):4410-5. doi:10.1073/pnas.1215927110.

Ragino YI, Stakhneva EM, Polonskaya YV, Kashtanova EV. The Role of Secretory Activity Molecules of Visceral Adipocytes in Abdominal Obesity in the Development of Cardiovascular Disease: A Review. *Biomolecules.* 2020 Feb 28;10(3). pii: E374. doi: 10.3390/biom10030374.

Ravera A, Carubelli V, Sciatti E, et al. Nutrition and Cardiovascular Disease: Finding the Perfect Recipe for Cardiovascular Health. *Nutrients.* 2016;8(6):363. Published 2016 Jun 14. doi: 10.3390/nu8060363.

Rocha NP, Milagres LC, Longo GZ, Ribeiro AQ, Novaes JF. Association between dietary pattern and cardiometabolic risk in children and adolescents: a systematic review. *J Pediatr (Rio J).* 2017;93(3):214–222. doi: 10.1016/j.jped.2017.01.002.

Ros E. Nuts and CVD. Br J Nutr. 2015;113 Suppl 2:S111–S120. doi: 10.1017/S0007114514003924.

Roshanravan N, Mahdavi R, Alizadeh E, Jafarabadi MA, Hedayati M, Ghavami A, Alipour S, Alamdari NM, Barati M, Ostadrahimi A. Effect of Butyrate and Inulin Supplementation on Glycemic Status, Lipid Profile and Glucagon-Like Peptide 1 Level in Patients with Type 2 Diabetes: A Randomized Double-Blind, Placebo-Controlled Trial. *Horm Metab Res*. 2017 Nov;49(11):886-891. doi: 10.1055/s-0043-119089.

Ruiz-Canela M, Bes-Rastrollo M, Martínez-González MA. The Role of Dietary Inflammatory Index in Cardiovascular Disease, Metabolic Syndrome and Mortality. *Int J Mol Sci*. 2016; 17(8):1265. Published 2016 Aug 3. doi: 10.3390/ijms17081265.

Ruiz-Canela M, Zazpe I, Shivappa N, et al. Dietary inflammatory index and anthropometric measures of obesity in a population sample at high cardiovascular risk from the PREDIMED (PREvención con DIeta MEDiterránea) trial. *Br J Nutr*. 2015;113(6):984–995. doi: 10.1017/S0007114514004401.

Saad MJ, Santos A, Prada PO. Linking Gut Microbiota and Inflammation to Obesity and Insulin Resistance. *Physiology (Bethesda)*. 2016 Jul;31(4):283-93. doi: 10.1152/physiol.00041.2015.

Sandek A, Bauditz J, Swidsinski A, Buhner S, Weber-Eibel J, von Haehling S, Schroedl W, Karhausen T, Doehner W, Rauchhaus M, Poole-Wilson P, Volk HD, Lochs H, Anker SD. Altered intestinal function in patients with chronic heart failure. *J Am Coll Cardiol*. 2007 Oct 16;50(16):1561-9.

Schwandt P, Haas GM, Bertsch T. Nutrition and Cardiovascular Risk Factors in Four Age Groups of Female Individuals: The PEP Family Heart Study. *Int J Prev Med*. 2010;1(2):103–109.

Schwingshackl L, Bogensberger B, Hoffmann G. Diet Quality as Assessed by the Healthy Eating Index, Alternate Healthy Eating Index, Dietary Approaches to Stop Hypertension Score, and Health Outcomes: An Updated Systematic Review and Meta-Analysis of Cohort Studies. *J Acad Nutr Diet*. 2018 Jan;118(1):74-100.e11. doi: 10.1016/j.jand.2017.08.024.

Schwingshackl L, Hoffmann G. Mediterranean dietary pattern, inflammation and endothelial function: a systematic review and meta-analysis of intervention trials. *Nutr Metab Cardiovasc Dis.* 2014; 24(9):929–939. doi:10.1016/j.numecd.2014.03.003.

Senthong V, Wang Z, Fan Y, Wu Y, Hazen SL, Tang WH. Trimethylamine N-Oxide and Mortality Risk in Patients With Peripheral Artery Disease. *J Am Heart Assoc.* 2016 Oct 19;5(10). pii: e004237.

Serino A, Salazar G. Protective Role of Polyphenols against Vascular Inflammation, Aging and Cardiovascular Disease. *Nutrients.* 2018;11(1):53. Published 2018 Dec 28. doi: 10.3390/nu11010053.

Shivappa N, Godos J, Hébert JR, et al. Dietary Inflammatory Index and Cardiovascular Risk and Mortality-A Meta-Analysis. *Nutrients.* 2018;10(2):200. Published 2018 Feb 12. doi: 10.3390/nu10020200.

Shivappa N, Steck SE, Hurley TG, Hussey JR, Hébert JR. Designing and developing a literature-derived, population-based dietary inflammatory index. *Public Health Nutr.* 2014;17(8):1689–1696. doi: 10.1017/S1368 980013002115.

Siervo M, Lara J, Chowdhury S, Ashor A, Oggioni C, Mathers JC. Effects of the Dietary Approach to Stop Hypertension (DASH) diet on cardiovascular risk factors: a systematic review and meta-analysis. *Br J Nutr.* 2015;113(1):1–15. doi: 10.1017/S0007114514003341.

Sima P, Vannucci L, Vetvicka V. β-glucans and cholesterol (Review). *Int J Mol Med.* 2018;41(4):1799–1808. doi:10.3892/ijmm.2018.3411.

Sofi F, Macchi C, Abbate R, Gensini GF, Casini A. Mediterranean diet and health status: an updated meta-analysis and a proposal for a literature-based adherence score. *Public Health Nutr.* 2014;17(12):2769–2782. doi: 10.1017/S1368980013003169.

Sozen E, Demirel T, Ozer NK. Vitamin E: Regulatory role in the cardiovascular system. *IUBMB Life.* 2019;71(4):507–515. doi: 10.1002/iub.2020.

Steyers CM 3rd, Miller FJ Jr. Endothelial dysfunction in chronic inflammatory diseases. *Int J Mol Sci.* 2014 Jun 25;15(7):11324-49. doi: 10.3390/ijms150711324.

Świątecka D, Narbad A, Ridgway KP, Kostyra H. The study on the impact of glycated pea proteins on human intestinal bacteria. *Int J Food Microbiol.* 2011 Jan 31;145(1):267-72. doi: 10.1016/j.ijfoodmicro. 2011.01.002.

Tandon P, Wafer R, Minchin JEN. Adipose morphology and metabolic disease. *J Exp Biol.* 2018 Mar 7;221(Pt Suppl 1). pii: jeb164970. doi: 10.1242/jeb.164970.

Tazoe H, Otomo Y, Karaki S, Kato I, Fukami Y, Terasaki M, Kuwahara A. Expression of short-chain fatty acid receptor GPR41 in the human colon. *Biomed Res.* 2009 Jun;30(3):149-56.

Tousoulis D, Plastiras A, Siasos G, et al. Omega-3 PUFAs improved endothelial function and arterial stiffness with a parallel antiinflammatory effect in adults with metabolic syndrome. *Atherosclerosis.* 2014; 232(1):10–16. doi:10.1016/j.atherosclerosis. 2013.10.014.

U.S. Department of Health and Human Services and U.S. Department of Agriculture. *2015–2020 Dietary Guidelines for Americans.* 8th Edition. December 2015. Available at http://health.gov/dietaryguidelines/2015/guidelines/.

Walker AW, Ince J, Duncan SH, Webster LM, Holtrop G, Ze X, Brown D, Stares MD, Scott P, Bergerat A, Louis P, McIntosh F, Johnstone AM, Lobley GE, Parkhill J, Flint HJ. Dominant and diet-responsive groups of bacteria within the human colonic microbiota. *ISME J.* 2011 Feb;5(2):220-30. doi: 10.1038/ismej.2010.118.

Wang Q, Liang X, Wang L, et al. Effect of omega-3 fatty acids supplementation on endothelial function: a meta-analysis of randomized controlled trials. *Atherosclerosis.* 2012;221(2):536–543. doi: 10.1016/j.atherosclerosis.2012.01.006.

Wang Z, Klipfell E, Bennett BJ, Koeth R, Levison BS, Dugar B, Feldstein AE, Britt EB, Fu X, Chung YM, Wu Y, Schauer P, Smith JD, Allayee H, Tang WH, DiDonato JA, Lusis AJ, Hazen SL. Gut flora metabolism of phosphatidylcholine promotes cardiovascular disease. *Nature.* 2011 Apr 7;472(7341):57-63. doi: 10.1038/nature09922.

Wilck N, Matus MG, Kearney SM, Olesen SW, Forslund K, Bartolomaeus H, Haase S, Mähler A, Balogh A, Markó L, Vvedenskaya O, Kleiner FH, Tsvetkov D, Klug L, Costea PI, Sunagawa S, Maier L, Rakova N, Schatz V, Neubert P, Frätzer C, Krannich A, Gollasch M, Grohme DA, Côrte-Real BF, Gerlach RG, Basic M, Typas A, Wu C, Titze JM, Jantsch J, Boschmann M, Dechend R, Kleinewietfeld M, Kempa S, Bork P, Linker RA, Alm EJ, Müller DN. Salt-responsive gut commensal modulates T(H)17 axis and disease. *Nature.* 2017 Nov 30;551(7682):585-589. doi: 10.1038/nature24628.

World Health Organization - WHO. *Obesity and overweight.* 2017 http://wwwwhoint/newsroom/fact-sheets/detail/obesity-and-overweight.

World Health Organization (WHO). *Disponível* em: <https://www.who.int/news-room/fact-sheets/detail/healthy-diet>. Acesso em: 10 de dezembro de 2019.

Yan H, Ajuwon KM. Butyrate modifies intestinal barrier function in IPEC-J2 cells through a selective upregulation of tight junction proteins and activation of the Akt signaling pathway. *PLoS One.* 2017 Jun 27;12(6):e0179586. doi: 10.1371/journal.pone.0179586.

Yang T, Santisteban MM, Rodriguez V, Li E, Ahmari N, Carvajal JM, Zadeh M, Gong M, Qi Y, Zubcevic J, Sahay B, Pepine CJ, Raizada MK, Mohamadzadeh M. Gut dysbiosis is linked to hypertension. *Hypertension.* 2015 Jun; 65(6):1331-40. doi: 10.1161/HYPERTEN SIONAHA.115.05315.

Zhong X, Guo L, Zhang L, Li Y, He R, Cheng G. Inflammatory potential of diet and risk of cardiovascular disease or mortality: A meta-analysis. *Sci Rep.* 2017;7(1):6367. Published 2017 Jul 25. doi:10.1038/s41598-017-06455-x.

Zhu W, Gregory JC, Org E, Buffa JA, Gupta N, Wang Z, Li L, Fu X, Wu Y, Mehrabian M, Sartor RB, McIntyre TM, Silverstein RL, Tang WHW, DiDonato JA, Brown JM, Lusis AJ, Hazen SL. Gut Microbial Metabolite TMAO Enhances Platelet Hyperreactivity and Thrombosis Risk. *Cell.* 2016 Mar 24; 165(1):111-124. doi: 10.1016/j.cell.2016.02.011.

INDEX

A

acid, 9, 23, 24, 27, 32, 33, 34, 37, 51, 89, 90, 94, 96, 99, 107, 108, 110, 114
adaptation(s), 67, 97, 106
adipocyte, 19, 29, 54, 55, 74, 76, 77, 90
adiponectin, 13, 19, 55, 56, 58, 74, 76, 91, 92
adipose, viii, 43, 45, 49, 53, 54, 55, 74, 75, 88, 89, 90, 91, 92, 99, 101, 102, 109
adipose tissue, viii, 43, 45, 49, 53, 54, 55, 74, 75, 88, 89, 90, 91, 92, 99, 101, 102, 109
adiposity, vii, 1, 2, 8, 12, 13, 18, 19, 35, 48, 49, 53, 55, 58, 59, 68, 73, 74, 75, 78, 89
adolescents, 25, 46, 50, 77, 96, 105, 111
adults, 20, 29, 30, 32, 38, 41, 57, 89, 114
advanced glycation end-products, 6
age, 2, 4, 13, 27, 31, 45, 48, 49, 50, 53, 57, 59, 61, 85, 89, 92
American Heart Association, 19, 78, 104
androgen, 44, 46, 48, 49, 54, 57, 58, 59, 61, 65, 67, 68, 75, 79
androgens, 54, 55, 57, 59, 74, 77, 80
antioxidant, 39, 59, 80, 93

apolipoprotein B (apo-B), 8, 9, 10, 21, 34, 36, 39, 51
artery, viii, 30, 44, 45, 56, 64, 91, 109
assessment, 17, 46, 53, 63, 65, 83
atherosclerosis, 3, 8, 10, 16, 26, 33, 45, 55, 61, 77, 90, 91, 93, 94, 99, 103, 107, 109, 114
atherosclerotic plaque, 93, 99, 100

B

bacteria, 97, 99, 100, 108, 114
beneficial effect, 6, 72, 94, 100, 102
binding globulin, 44, 48, 54, 68
biomarkers, 25, 95, 96, 105, 106
blood, 3, 5, 6, 12, 14, 15, 17, 18, 20, 26, 28, 38, 49, 52, 54, 56, 58, 60, 73, 79, 90, 91, 92, 93, 94, 95, 97, 99, 100, 110, 111
blood pressure, 12, 17, 26, 28, 49, 52, 56, 60, 73, 79, 90, 92, 93, 94, 95, 99, 110, 111
BMI, 13, 15, 48, 49, 50, 51, 52, 53, 57, 58, 59, 89, 98
body fat, viii, 53, 55, 78, 88
body mass index, 8, 13, 23, 78, 81, 89
body weight, 22, 71, 88

Index

Brazil, viii, 87, 88

C

calcification(s), 45, 56, 64, 90
calcium, viii, 44, 100
carbohydrates, 90, 94, 98
cardio vascular diseases (CVD)
cardio vascular diseases (CVD), 2, 3, 4, 5, 8, 10, 13, 15, 25, 44, 51, 54, 57, 58, 60, 69, 94, 97, 98, 99, 100, 101, 102, 111
cardio-metabolic risk factors, vii, viii, 44, 55
cardiomyopathy, 3, 24, 40
cardiovascular disease(s) (CVD), vii, viii, 1, 2, 3, 4, 5, 8, 10, 12, 13, 14, 15, 18, 19, 20, 21, 22, 23, 25, 27, 28, 29, 30, 31, 33, 37, 38, 44, 45, 46, 51, 54, 55, 57, 58, 59, 60, 69, 71, 76, 77, 78, 79, 80, 82, 83, 85, 88, 89, 91, 92, 93, 94, 95, 96, 97, 98, 99, 100, 101, 102, 104, 105, 108, 111, 114, 115
cardiovascular risk, vii, viii, 3, 6, 7, 8, 9, 10, 13, 14, 16, 17, 22, 24, 25, 26, 28, 40, 45, 49, 53, 56, 59, 61, 72, 83, 84, 88, 89, 91, 92, 94, 96, 102, 103, 106, 109, 112, 113
central obesity, viii, 13, 15, 28, 44, 45, 52, 53, 54, 56, 57, 74, 110
Chicago, 7, 12, 13, 23, 33, 41
children, 25, 105, 111
cholesterol, 7, 8, 9, 10, 13, 14, 15, 17, 19, 20, 21, 22, 23, 27, 28, 30, 34, 35, 36, 37, 38, 39, 40, 51, 59, 91, 93, 94, 96, 98, 100, 104, 113
clustering, 14, 16, 18, 40
colon, 97, 98, 101, 106, 114
community, ix, 62, 65, 88
complications, 23, 26, 39, 64, 90, 92
composition, 33, 94, 97, 101, 102, 103
confounders, 50, 51, 62
consensus, 14, 19, 45, 46, 65, 105
consumption, 93, 101, 103, 106, 109, 110
controlled trials, 61, 94, 109, 114
coronary artery disease, 3, 4, 8, 11, 34, 38, 79
coronary heart disease, 3, 5, 12, 13, 15, 19, 23, 24, 27, 28, 30, 32, 33, 34, 35, 37, 38, 40, 75, 93, 101, 103, 107, 111
CRP, 58, 60, 82, 90, 96
cytokines, 29, 54, 56, 58, 60, 93, 98

D

deaths, 2, 3, 93
deficiency, 60, 61, 67, 84, 101
diabetes, viii, 2, 3, 4, 5, 6, 7, 8, 12, 13, 14, 15, 18, 19, 20, 21, 22, 23, 24, 25, 26, 28, 29, 30, 31, 32, 33, 34, 35, 36, 37, 38, 39, 41, 44, 46, 48, 49, 55, 60, 64, 67, 70, 73, 77, 84, 85, 94, 101, 102, 104, 109, 110, 111, 112
diabetes mellitus, 4, 20, 24, 26, 28, 29, 30, 31, 32, 33, 35, 37, 38, 40, 70, 73, 94, 102
diabetic patients, 5, 34, 39
diagnostic criteria, 45, 51, 63, 65
diet, ix, 48, 59, 88, 89, 90, 92, 93, 94, 95, 96, 97, 98, 100, 101, 102, 105, 106, 108, 109, 110, 113, 114, 115
diseases, viii, 2, 19, 29, 33, 38, 44, 55, 77, 82, 88, 89, 92, 93, 94, 95, 102, 103, 108
dyslipidemia, viii, 35, 44, 47, 50, 51, 56, 59, 71, 78, 79, 88, 94

E

electronegatively charged LDL (LDL^{-ve}), 8, 16, 18
endocrine, viii, 43, 44, 46, 47, 54, 61, 63, 88, 90
endocrinology, 65, 66, 68, 70, 71, 73, 74, 79, 80, 81, 82, 85
endothelial cells, 3, 22, 32, 91

endothelial dysfunction, viii, 3, 6, 9, 11, 12, 13, 18, 28, 32, 35, 44, 52, 56, 57, 58, 80, 81, 93, 105
endothelium, 30, 33, 37, 39, 52, 75, 99
energy, 47, 54, 55, 88, 89, 92, 97, 98, 101, 108
environment, 67, 84, 99
enzyme, 19, 72, 100
epidemic, viii, 41, 87, 88
epidemiology, 37, 62, 110
etiology, viii, 43, 44, 47, 67, 88
evidence, viii, 5, 6, 12, 25, 30, 40, 43, 50, 51, 52, 53, 54, 55, 59, 60, 72, 79, 93, 102, 105, 110
exercise, 69, 72, 76

F

fasting, 3, 4, 15, 17, 23, 49, 56, 60, 100
fasting glucose, 4, 15, 49, 56, 60
fat, 23, 33, 41, 53, 54, 59, 69, 74, 89, 93, 94, 95, 96, 97, 99, 100, 101, 102, 103, 104, 105, 106, 107, 109
fatty acids, vii, 1, 11, 13, 16, 18, 34, 36, 89, 90, 94, 96, 98, 104, 110, 114
fiber, 93, 101, 103
fibrinogen, 7, 20, 34, 35
fibrinolytic, 7, 59, 83
financial burden, 2
food, 96, 97, 101, 103
Ford, 4, 25, 30
formation, 10, 45, 83, 90, 100

G

gene expression, 55, 57, 66
genes, 47, 51, 60, 66, 67
glucose, viii, 3, 4, 5, 6, 13, 14, 15, 17, 18, 20, 27, 33, 34, 36, 37, 38, 44, 49, 50, 57, 60, 66, 68, 69, 70, 73, 91, 92, 99, 100, 102

glucose tolerance, 3, 4, 15, 17, 49, 50, 66, 70, 73
glucose tolerance test, 3, 17, 50
guidelines, 12, 65, 114

H

health, viii, 2, 11, 16, 18, 24, 31, 53, 62, 65, 76, 80, 84, 92, 94, 95, 102, 105, 107, 110, 113, 114
heart disease, 3, 5, 24, 33, 34, 36, 73, 85
heart failure, 2, 5, 75, 97, 100
high blood pressure, 17, 72, 91
high-density lipoprotein (HDL), vii, 1, 9, 10, 11, 14, 15, 16, 17, 18, 19, 20, 21, 22, 23, 24, 27, 32, 34, 36, 37, 39, 50, 51, 56, 57, 60, 91, 94
history, 50, 52, 62
homeostasis, 17, 47, 49, 54, 60, 92, 97
hormone(s0, 44, 46, 47, 48, 54, 55, 68, 108
host, 97, 99, 100, 101, 102
human, 23, 30, 32, 58, 60, 82, 83, 97, 101, 108, 110, 114
hyperandrogenemia, viii, 43, 44, 46, 49, 61
hyperandrogenism, 44, 45, 46, 48, 50, 52, 54, 57, 58, 66, 67, 68, 69, 75, 78, 79, 82, 83
hyperinsulinaemia, vii, 1, 2, 3, 13, 18
hyperinsulinemia, 30, 49, 52, 54, 55, 61
hypertension, viii, 11, 12, 23, 24, 25, 26, 27, 30, 33, 37, 38, 39, 40, 41, 44, 52, 53, 54, 56, 57, 69, 72, 73, 75, 79, 80, 93, 99, 109, 112, 113, 115
hypertrigliceridaemia, 10
hypertriglyceridemia, 51
hypertrophy, 3, 12, 13, 52, 54, 90, 91, 92, 97

I

immune system, 60, 97, 99

impaired glucose tolerance, 4, 15, 49, 70, 73
in vivo, 30, 40, 100
incidence, 12, 52, 70, 94
individuals, ix, 13, 17, 30, 88, 90, 91, 96, 99
induction, 9, 32, 51
inflammation, 6, 13, 17, 18, 20, 24, 25, 33, 41, 45, 47, 49, 54, 55, 57, 58, 59, 63, 75, 80, 82, 90, 93, 95, 98, 100, 102, 105, 107, 110, 113
inhibitor, 3, 7, 59, 92
injury, 12, 16, 26
insulin, vii, viii, 1, 3, 8, 9, 10, 11, 12, 13, 15, 17, 18, 20, 23, 25, 26, 27, 28, 31, 32, 37, 38, 41, 43, 44, 46, 47, 48, 50, 52, 54, 55, 56, 58, 59, 60, 66, 68, 71, 72, 73, 74, 76, 77, 78, 81, 82, 83, 89, 91, 92, 93, 94, 101, 102, 106, 107
insulin resistance, vii, viii, 1, 2, 3, 10, 11, 12, 13, 15, 17, 18, 20, 23, 25, 26, 28, 29, 32, 41, 43, 44, 46, 47, 48, 49, 50, 52, 55, 56, 58, 59, 60, 63, 66, 67, 68, 69, 71, 72, 73, 74, 76, 77, 78, 81, 82, 83, 85, 91, 92, 93, 94, 106, 112
insulin sensitivity, 17, 31, 32, 102
insulin signaling, 27, 37, 101
intervention, 2, 47, 113
intestine, 97, 99, 100
intima, viii, 8, 44, 45, 56, 64
issues, viii, 44, 62

L

later life, viii, 44, 53, 62
LDL, 8, 9, 10, 14, 16, 18, 21, 24, 25, 30, 39, 40, 50, 51, 57, 60, 91, 94
lead, 18, 48, 49, 52, 54
leptin, 55, 56, 76, 77, 89, 92
lipid metabolism, 54, 60, 71, 99
lipids, 53, 58, 84, 90, 91, 103, 109
lipolysis, 45, 51, 69, 89, 103

lipoproteins, 8, 9, 10, 28, 32, 38, 100, 103, 109
liver, viii, 11, 49, 88, 100, 101
low-density lipoprotein, 8, 91
low-density lipoprotein (LDL), vii, 1, 8, 9, 10, 14, 16, 18, 19, 21, 22, 24, 25, 27, 28, 29, 30, 38, 39, 40, 50, 51, 57, 60, 71, 91, 94
low-grade inflammation, 49, 54, 64, 104
Lp(a), 9, 22, 25

M

macrophages, 41, 89, 91
management, viii, 24, 38, 44, 62, 78, 80, 104
mass, viii, 20, 53, 55, 88, 92, 97, 102
meat, 93, 100, 107
media, viii, 8, 44, 45, 56, 64
medicine, 64, 71, 82
Mediterranean, 93, 96, 113
mellitus, 4, 20, 24, 26, 28, 29, 30, 31, 32, 33, 35, 37, 38, 40, 70, 73, 94, 102
menopause, 52, 61, 63
meta-analysis, 3, 4, 5, 8, 14, 19, 21, 22, 24, 25, 27, 29, 50, 52, 53, 55, 57, 60, 61, 63, 64, 68, 70, 71, 73, 74, 76, 77, 79, 80, 82, 83, 84, 85, 94, 106, 109, 113, 114, 115
Metabolic, v, vii, 1, 14, 23, 25, 40, 43, 48, 56, 57, 74, 75, 79, 81, 104, 105, 108, 110, 112
metabolic disorder, viii, 43, 65, 88, 90, 92
metabolic disturbances, 47, 50, 54, 56, 60, 61, 83
metabolic health, viii, 2, 11, 16, 18, 24
metabolic syndrome, viii, 7, 8, 11, 12, 14, 15, 17, 18, 19, 21, 23, 25, 26, 28, 29, 30, 33, 34, 40, 44, 46, 53, 55, 56, 57, 70, 72, 73, 74, 75, 78, 79, 84, 88, 93, 102, 107, 110, 114
metabolically healthy normal weight, 17

Index

metabolically healthy obese, 17
metabolically unhealthy normal weight, 17
metabolically unhealthy obese, 17
metabolism, ix, 34, 38, 58, 65, 67, 69, 70, 71, 74, 80, 81, 84, 88, 92, 97, 99, 102, 107, 110, 114
metabolites, 90, 98, 110
mice, 83, 101, 102
microbiota, 91, 97, 98, 99, 100, 101, 102, 107, 109, 110, 111, 114
morbidity, vii, 1, 47, 89
morphology, 44, 45, 46, 74, 114
mortality, vii, 1, 2, 3, 4, 5, 6, 7, 11, 12, 13, 19, 20, 21, 22, 23, 24, 26, 27, 28, 29, 30, 31, 34, 37, 39, 40, 41, 42, 45, 89, 93, 96, 97, 103, 108, 115
myocardial infarction, 2, 4, 5, 9, 10, 13, 24, 27, 28, 29, 32, 33, 39, 41, 42, 96, 100

N

National Health and Nutrition Examination Survey, 17, 30, 103
nitric oxide, 32, 33, 37, 52, 58, 91
nutrient(s), 95, 97, 100, 102, 107, 108
nutrition, ix, 48, 88
nutritional habits, vii, ix, 88

O

obesity, v, viii, 8, 11, 12, 13, 14, 15, 17, 19, 20, 21, 22, 23, 24, 25, 27, 28, 29, 30, 31, 37, 38, 41, 44, 45, 46, 47, 48, 50, 52, 53, 54, 55, 56, 57, 58, 59, 62, 63, 64, 65, 70, 72, 74, 75, 76, 79, 81, 83, 87, 88, 89, 90, 91, 92, 93, 94, 96, 97, 98, 101, 102, 103, 104, 105, 106, 107, 108, 109, 110, 111, 112, 115
omega-3, 93, 95, 114
overweight, 17, 29, 53, 57, 75, 89, 104, 109, 115

oxidative stress, 6, 18, 26, 35, 45, 57, 58, 59, 64, 71, 75, 80, 81, 82, 83, 93, 99, 100
oxidised LDL, 8, 18

P

participants, 27, 35, 41, 97
pathogenesis, vii, viii, 1, 18, 37, 43, 44, 58, 60, 71
pathophysiology, 58, 59, 64, 72
pathway(s), ix, 3, 6, 16, 23, 27, 47, 48, 49, 56, 88, 91, 93, 98, 100
peptide(s), 3, 6, 31, 32, 49, 54, 55, 69, 70, 101
permeability, 98, 100, 103
pharmaceutical, 64, 65, 75
phenotype(s), 39, 40, 46, 48, 51, 57, 63, 65, 66, 67, 68, 81, 84, 85
physiology, 72, 77, 83
placebo, 12, 22, 26
plaque, 56, 91, 107
plasminogen, 3, 7, 19, 59, 92
platelet aggregation, 59, 90, 101
PM, 22, 27, 28, 63, 72, 108
policy, vii, viii, 44
policy makers, vii, viii, 44
polycystic ovarian syndrome, 64, 68, 72, 76, 77, 83, 84
polycystic ovary syndrome (PCOS), vii, viii, 43, 44, 45, 46, 47, 48, 49, 50, 51, 52, 53, 54, 55, 56, 57, 58, 59, 60, 61, 62, 63, 64, 65, 66, 67, 68, 69, 70, 71, 72, 73, 74, 75, 76, 77, 78, 79, 80, 81, 82, 83, 84, 85
polymorphism(s), 48, 55, 66, 68, 76, 81, 84
polyol pathway, 6, 23
polyphenols, 93, 101, 107
population, vii, viii, 2, 7, 11, 13, 23, 31, 37, 40, 44, 49, 51, 52, 57, 58, 59, 61, 62, 63, 67, 70, 73, 81, 87, 92, 93, 112, 113
progenitor cell, 6, 11, 35, 36
prognosis, 8, 58, 104

pro-inflammatory, viii, 9, 39, 60, 84, 88, 89, 90, 91, 92, 96, 98
protein kinase C, 6, 29, 37
proteins, 58, 66, 98, 114, 115
public health, vii, 1, 2

R

receptor(s), 3, 22, 32, 48, 49, 51, 55, 60, 66, 69, 83, 84, 89, 91, 98, 99, 102, 107, 108, 110, 111, 114
recommendations, iv, vii, viii, 44, 75
regression, 70, 73, 74, 109
relevance, 23, 24, 92
renin, 52, 54, 57, 80, 99, 111
reproduction, 54, 63, 64, 65, 68, 70, 73, 74, 76, 78, 82
reproductive age, 44, 52, 61
resistance, vii, viii, 1, 3, 7, 10, 11, 12, 13, 17, 18, 20, 23, 25, 26, 28, 32, 41, 43, 44, 46, 47, 48, 49, 50, 52, 54, 55, 56, 58, 59, 60, 63, 66, 67, 68, 69, 71, 72, 73, 74, 76, 77, 78, 81, 82, 83, 85, 91, 92, 93, 94, 106
response, 30, 39, 59, 60, 69
risk(s), vii, viii, ix, 3, 4, 5, 6, 7, 8, 9, 10, 11, 12, 13, 14, 17, 19, 20, 21, 23, 24, 25, 27, 28, 32, 33, 34, 35, 37, 39, 40, 41, 42, 44, 45, 47, 49, 51, 52, 53, 54, 55, 56, 57, 59, 60, 61, 62, 63, 67, 70, 71, 73, 75, 78, 79, 80, 82, 83, 85, 88, 89, 91, 92, 93, 94, 95, 96, 97, 98, 99, 100, 101, 102, 103, 104, 105, 107, 111, 115
risk factors, vii, viii, ix, 4, 11, 14, 37, 42, 44, 45, 55, 61, 62, 67, 70, 73, 79, 83, 85, 88, 91, 104

S

saturated fat, 93, 94, 101, 102, 109
scope, viii, 2, 4, 44

secretion, 44, 49, 54, 55, 61, 77, 90, 93, 99, 101, 111
senescence, 9, 11, 36, 40
serum, 7, 9, 11, 14, 17, 33, 37, 38, 51, 55, 60, 63, 74, 76, 77, 84, 94, 100, 109
sex, 44, 48, 54, 68, 74
signaling pathway, 36, 51, 115
smooth muscle, 10, 90, 103
sodium, 6, 52, 93, 110
state, viii, 7, 16, 17, 38, 58, 73, 75, 88, 90, 91
states, 3, 8, 11
statin, 7, 10, 21
stress, 6, 18, 26, 35, 45, 57, 58, 59, 64, 71, 75, 80, 81, 82, 83, 91, 93, 99, 100
stroke, 5, 8, 24, 33, 35, 40, 83, 100, 105
substrate, 3, 32, 48, 98
Sun, 25, 68, 72, 77, 84
supplementation, 61, 84, 95, 99
syndrome, vii, viii, 7, 8, 11, 12, 14, 15, 17, 18, 19, 21, 23, 25, 26, 28, 29, 30, 33, 34, 40, 43, 44, 45, 46, 47, 52, 53, 54, 55, 56, 57, 62, 63, 64, 65, 66, 67, 68, 69, 70, 71, 72, 73, 74, 75, 76, 77, 78, 79, 80, 81, 82, 83, 84, 85, 88, 93, 102, 107, 110, 114
synthesis, 32, 97, 98

T

testosterone, 48, 54, 57, 66, 68
therapy, 12, 19, 22, 40, 72, 96
thrombosis, 24, 64, 83
tissue, 20, 49, 53, 54, 63, 64, 74, 89, 90
TNF, 13, 49, 54, 58, 89, 90, 92, 96
TNF-α, 13, 49, 54, 58, 89, 90, 96
transport, 10, 19, 100
treatment, 12, 15, 24, 26, 27, 39, 40, 51, 59, 61, 63, 64, 66, 74, 76, 80, 101
trial, 6, 12, 22, 26, 27, 35, 38, 40, 69, 112
triglycerides, 11, 14, 15, 16, 17, 22, 26, 33, 36, 56, 90, 94, 95, 100

Index

type 2 diabetes, 4, 5, 8, 10, 15, 18, 21, 22, 23, 25, 26, 27, 28, 29, 30, 33, 35, 39, 40, 42, 70, 84

vitamin D, 60, 66, 83, 84, 85, 94
vitamin D deficiency, 60, 83, 84
VLDL, 30, 50, 51

U

ultrasound, 4, 8, 33, 46
United Kingdom, viii, 5, 38, 88
United States, viii, 17, 87, 109

W

weight loss, 75, 81, 91
World Health Organization (WHO), viii, 13, 14, 15, 30, 33, 41, 87, 89, 101, 109, 115
worldwide, 2, 13, 19

V

variations, 46, 48, 89
vascular diseases, 44
visceral adiposity, 49, 53, 55, 78

Y

young women, 50, 71, 79, 80, 81